I0090255

Ayurveda

The Ayurveda Book for Self-healing and Detoxification

(Essential Ayurvedic Principles and Practices to Balance and Heal Naturally)

Henry Barber

Published By **Chris David**

Henry Barber

All Rights Reserved

Ayurveda: The Ayurveda Book for Self-healing and Detoxification (Essential Ayurvedic Principles and Practices to Balance and Heal Naturally)

ISBN 978-1-7777786-5-1

No part of this guidebook shall be reproduced in any form without permission in writing from the publisher except in the case of brief quotations embodied in critical articles or reviews.

Legal & Disclaimer

The information contained in this book is not designed to replace or take the place of any form of medicine or professional medical advice. The information in this book has been provided for educational & entertainment purposes only.

The information contained in this book has been compiled from sources deemed reliable, and it is accurate to the best of the Author's knowledge; however, the Author cannot guarantee its accuracy and validity and cannot be held liable for any errors or omissions. Changes are periodically made to this book. You must consult your doctor or get professional medical advice before using any of the suggested remedies, techniques, or information in this book.

Upon using the information contained in this book, you agree to hold harmless the Author from and against any damages, costs, and expenses, including any legal fees potentially resulting from the application of any of the information provided by this guide. This disclaimer applies to any damages or injury caused by the use and application, whether directly or indirectly, of any advice or information presented, whether for breach of contract, tort, negligence, personal injury, criminal intent, or under any other cause of action.

You agree to accept all risks of using the information presented inside this book. You need to consult a professional medical practitioner in order to ensure you are both able and healthy enough to participate in this program.

Table Of Contents

Chapter 1: Ayurveda For The Modern Woman

SIMPLIFYING ANCIENT WISDOM

In this fast-paced society the ancient wisdom of Ayurveda may seem far-fetched and obscure. However, its wisdom, which is rooted in years of study and experience can provide effective solutions to the current problems. The trick is to distill the essence of it, and so that it is accessible and useful to the modern woman. Today, women are juggling roles whether as professional or caregivers, partners or even parents, they frequently have to deal with imbalance, stress and an inability to connect with their true selves. Imagine if the vast knowledge that is Ayurveda could be distilled into concrete knowledge? The insights seamlessly integrate with our modern-day lifestyles without too overwhelming?

REDISCOVERING THE BASICS

The essence of Ayurveda is about self-knowledge by focusing on the body's messages, and having a harmonious relationship with nature. It's not about elaborate practices or inaccessible herbs. Instead, it's about making small daily options. Selecting foods that match your constitution and allowing time for reflection and recognizing one's own natural rhythms.

A TIME-TESTED GUIDE IN A DIGITAL AGE

In an age of digital technology and rapid information access, Ayurveda offers the wisdom from the past. It's not to say that it's obsolete. Consider it as a reliable guide that offers time-tested tips to meet the demands of modern times. It doesn't matter if it's fighting screen-induced eyestrain or finding a way to find mental tranquility amid the constant stream of messages, Ayurveda provides solutions that have stood the testing of the test of.

BRIDGING THE OLD WITH THE NEW

The incorporation of Ayurveda into our modern lives doesn't necessarily mean sacrificing modern conveniences or innovations. It's all about integration. Utilizing Ayurvedic herbs to supplement your regular food regimen, doing yoga as part of a routine exercise routine, or utilizing applications for meditation to bring mindfulness into your daily routine. The key is to find the equilibrium that is most beneficial for an person.

THE FLEXIBILITY OF AYURVEDA

One of the advantages of Ayurveda is its flexibility. Though the principles are consistent however, the way they are applied can differ. An over-worked mother may be able to relax with a five-minute meditation in her lunch break and a professional could benefit from tailored eating habits to help combat work stress. Ayurveda has a wide range of treatments and methods is able to be tailored to suit the modern woman's particular requirements. Ayurveda specifically for modern women can be described as making its wealth easy to access, practical and useful. It's about gaining its immense advantages without being overwhelmed making sure that everyone regardless of her life style is able to walk in the direction to health, balance, and inner peace.

ADAPTING AYURVEDA TO URBAN LIVING

The urban lifestyle, with its high-rises, tightly scheduled schedules as well as the constant buzz of activity It can be a far cry far from the tranquil nature and serene ashrams commonly connected with Ayurveda. However, Ayurvedic principles don't have to be tied to any specific place; they're adaptable and flexible. Find out how to integrate the wisdom and tradition of Ayurveda to meet the demands and the nuances of urban living.

FINDING NATURE AMIDST CONCRETE

Although cities are mostly filled with concrete There are still places of natural beauty that are waiting to be explored. These include the city park, rooftop garden or even indoor plants they can become a haven. Walking in parks regularly or establishing a tiny backyard garden will help you stay connected to the natural world, and help you breathe in fresh air and take in some the peace and tranquility of your day.

MEAL PREPPING WITH AYURVEDIC PRINCIPLES

The hustle and bustle of urban living, eating take-outs or processed food items has become the norm for many. But with a little some planning Ayurvedic dishes can be integrated within busy lifestyles. Set aside a time each Saturday to make nutritious, dosha-specific dishes to prepare for the coming week. With the help of local items, Ayurvedic cooking can be healthy and easy to prepare.

MINDFUL BREAKS IN A BUSY DAY

The modern lifestyle is a synonym for productivity and busyness, Ayurveda stresses the importance of taking breaks and mindfulness. Easy practices like meditation exercises that allow you to breathe deeply during your commute or short meditations in lunch breaks, or even exercises that focus on grounding, like touching the surface of your desk help you bring moments of calm and refueling your body into the day.

DIGITAL DETOX AND SLEEP HYGIENE

The enticement of screen devices, from phones to laptops, increases when you live in urban areas. However, Ayurveda stresses the importance of rest and the equilibrium between relaxation and activity. Making sure you have a screen-free time before bedtime, establishing an environment that promotes sleep with soft light and soft sounds as well as prioritizing your sleep time can make the world of difference for the quality of your life.

COMMUNITY AND GROUP PRACTICES

The cities often have a variety of activities for groups. From meditation classes, yoga and yoga classes to Ayurvedic cooking courses There's an activity that is suitable for all. Involving in group exercises will not only boost your motivation, but also create connections among like-minded persons, and create feelings of belonging as well as mutual growth. The urban lifestyle, though demanding, should not cause a problem for practicing Ayurveda. Through small, mindful changes and choices that rely on the wisdom of Ayurveda is able to become an integral and beneficial part of an urban woman's lifestyle, leading her to balance, wellness and peace of mind in the chaos of city life.

OVERCOMING MODERN-DAY CHALLENGES WITH AYURVEDA

We get it. The way we live today isn't as easy as it was. Our fast-paced life in has a myriad of problems such as anxiety, stress with endless tasks to complete as well as the sense that the hours of a day do not suffice. However, there's a bright side: Ayurveda has got your back.

STRESS AND BURNOUT

Today, stress is like that unwanted guest who will not leave. But, thanks to Ayurveda you can find a way to get rid of stress. Instead of reaching for the three-cup of caffeinated coffee consider sipping warm, spicy milk. This is a straightforward switch that could do wonders for your mood. If work is wearing your body out? Take a few short breaks. Get up, stretch out or just look through the windows. Just a few minutes of silence will recharge you faster than you realize.

LACK OF SLEEP

Do you find yourself tossing and turning while in bed? Ayurveda recommends that a regular routine may be a game changer. Relax by turning off devices an hour before going to bed. You can instead read a book or relax with music. Simple tweaks, big results.

DIGESTIVE ISSUES

With the abundance of food choices available and the urge to go for fast food that our stomachs usually take the most of the burden. If you're feeling unbalanced or just feeling a bit off, Ayurveda suggests drinking hot water accompanied by a squeeze of lemon. Try eating your meals according to a regular schedule. The stomach is a lover of predictability.

FEELING DISCONNECTED

In the midst of endless messages, it's easy to become disconnected from your surroundings. Ayurveda's advice? Take a few minutes to be alone each day. This might be a brief stroll, a peaceful period with a cup tea or taking a deep breath. This is like having a date with your self. The great thing about Ayurveda is it doesn't require for huge drastic adjustments. The focus is on the little adjustments - the small changes which can result in big shifts. Therefore, in the chaos of our times be aware that Ayurveda provides simple, practical solutions. Take a deep breath, and then take the first step.

TOOLS AND TECHNIQUES FOR EVERYDAY LIFE

Life in the modern world can be an endless stream of obligations engagements, obligations, and distractions. In the midst of all this what can we do to achieve the balance? Below are a few Ayurvedic strategies and methods that are broken down into detail for you to navigate every day life effortlessly and with grace.

BALANCING DAILY ROUTINES WITH DINACHARYA

Dinacharya is referring to the Ayurvedic everyday routine, highlighting how important it is to have regularity throughout our life. How can adjust to this environment that's dominated by unreliable routines?

Start your day early: Ayurveda suggests rising with the sun. Although 5 am may be too much for some people who are not used to it, you can set your alarm thirty minutes later than normal. It is a time of peace that can be a time for reflection or for a relaxing morning walk.

Tongue Cleaning: An easy device that is known as a tongue scraper and available online or in the wellness shops, should be employed early in the morning. The practice isn't just about the hygiene of your mouth but, according to Ayurveda it also assists in removing any toxins built up over the night.

self-massage (Abhyanga): A quick five-minute massage at the beginning of your day by using warm sesame or coconut oil could stimulate circulation, and soothe your nervous system. This is like giving yourself the ultimate spa treatment prior to when your day begins!

EATING FOR BALANCE

Food isn't just about filling up our stomachs. It's about providing nourishment to our entire body. However, with errands, meetings and other chores, how do keep a healthy eating plan?

Mindful eating: Even during the busiest of days try to consume at least one meal in a quiet environment. Turn off the television and put the phone down and take the time to enjoy each bite. In the case of lunch breaks at work locate a peaceful spot, or meet a coworker to have a pleasant conversation, and not talk about the work.

Warm Breakfasts: Switch out the cold cereals and opt for something warmer, such as oatmeal that is topped with seasonal fruits or a delicious porridge of vegetables. Warm foods are more easy to digest and provide a warm start to your morning.

MANAGING STRESS

Life can throw up curveballs. It's just a fact. However, Ayurveda provides some useful instruments to help you catch them, without being overwhelmed.

Chapter 2: Embracing The Monthly Cycle

UNDERSTANDING THE MENSTRUAL CYCLE THROUGH AYURVEDA

Women have been taught to think of menstrual cycles as a burden or nuisance. However, Ayurveda reveres this natural menstrual cycle and views it as a potent detoxification process and an indicator of women's general health and energy. So let's explore the Ayurvedic view to understand the intricate details of the menstrual cycle.

NATURE'S RHYTHM WITHIN YOU

In Ayurveda the whole system is interconnected and the natural rhythms are replicated in our body. As the moon affects the water, its cycles affect the reproductive system of females. Do you have any experience of the menstrual cycle of your body synchronizing to the lunar phase? Women often menstruate during the new moon, and also ovulate at when the moon is full. This is testimony to our body's connection to the cosmic.

DOSHAS AND MENSTRUATION

Ayurveda believes that the body are controlled by three main Doshas or energies: Vata, Pitta as well as Kapha. The doshas also play a function in the menstrual cycle.

Vata: This type of dosha is the dominant one in the weeks leading up to menstrual. It's characterised by movement and space. It's the reason for the common issues of anxiety, bloating and insecurity that many women feel during in the pre-period.

Pitta Dosha: This fiery one governs the time of blood flow. Imagine the intense heat and intensity of menstrual flow: the irritation as well as the cramps and the intense emotional reactions. This is Pitta active.

Kapha Menstrual cycle: Following menstrual cycles which leads to the Ovulation, Kapha's earthy the qualities of water come to the picture. You feel a greater sense of peace and security physical, as your body is preparing to become pregnant, holding more fluids and constructing the inner lining of the uterus.

THE FOUR PHASES OF THE CYCLE

The menstrual cycle doesn't have to be just focused on the handful of periods of bleeding. It's an entire month of hormonal changes and physiological shifts. Through the perspective of an Ayurvedic lens, the cycle is seen through four sections:

1. Menstrual Period (Day 1-5) In this phase, the body eliminates the Uterine Line. It's a time to purify and release emotional and physically. Ayurveda recommends taking the time to relax during this period and giving your body the relaxation it needs.

2. Follicular Phase (Day 6 - 14) post menstrual period The body prepares itself to ovulate. The hormone estrogen is soaring and makes many women feel more energetic and social. Ayurvedically this is an ideal moment to be creative and make plans.

3. Ovulatory Phase (Day 14-17) A woman releases eggs from the Ovaries. The next few days may see the increase of libido as well as confidence due to an increase in hormone levels.

4. Luteal Phase (Day 18-28) When there is no fertilization of the egg, your body is preparing for the removal of the lining of the uterus. Progesterone levels increase in the uterus, and there is an urge to contemplation or nesting.

DIET AND LIFESTYLE CHANGES FOR A PAIN-FREE PERIOD

Menstrual flow is an innate process However, for a lot of women, it can cause uncomfortableness, pain as well as emotional turbulence. Ayurveda is a holistic approach, gives valuable insight regarding lifestyle and dietary changes that will significantly ease problems with menstruation. Let's look into some of the methods that help women toward a more peaceful and a more harmonious menstrual cycle.

FOOD THAT NOURISHES AND COMFORTS

Ayurveda holds the power of food to heal especially when it comes to menstrual cycles, the correct diet could do wonders.

1. Warm, cooked and warm meals Foods that are cold can boost Vata dosha levels, which can lead to greater cramps. Choose warmer, easy-to-digest meals. Consider stews, soups, and steaming vegetables.

2. Spices to Balance: Include spice blends like cumin, fennel as well as ginger. They not only aid in digestion, they also bring warmth neutralizing the coolness menstrual cycles.

3. Hydration in a Twist drinking enough water is vital and you should drink hot water, herbal teas or warm drinks. The addition of lemon juice or honey will also aid in cleansing and bringing the feeling of comfort.

4. Do not drink too much sugar or caffeine as both can trigger menstrual cramps. Instead of caffeine, consider the herbal tea, or warm

milk mixed with a little turmeric to boost your energy levels.

LIFESTYLE HABITS FOR HARMONY

It's not only about food choices however, it's also about the way you live. Here are a few Ayurvedic life tips to have an easy and painless period

1. Keep Warm: This cannot be overemphasized enough. Warm temperatures ease Vata disturbances. Also, make sure you wrap yourself with warm blankets, put on socks and stay away from the cold.

2. Gentle exercise: Though vigorous workouts may cause cramps, gentle exercise such as yoga are extremely advantageous. Poses like the child's pose the forward bend and butterfly pose are particularly comforting during menstrual cycles.

3. Abdominal Massages: With the warm oil of sesame or another Ayurvedic herb oil, massage gently your lower abdominal area. It

is not just helpful to ease cramps, but helps to build a stronger relationship to the body.

4. Make time for rest: Your body is going through major changes; you're bound to feel exhausted. Be aware of your body's needs and take a good night's sleep. Short naps, or even relaxing for a short time can help you reenergize.

5. Practice breathing and meditation exercises Help in calming and grounding the mind. Particularly when the emotions are up, a couple of minutes of meditation or deep breathing could make a world of change.

A Practical Example: Picture you're on the first day of your period and you're experiencing those familiar cramps starting to set in. Instead of seeking painkillers You decide to go for the Ayurvedic method. It is a simple vegetable soup that is seasoned with ginger and cumin. When it is simmering in the pot, you take part in a quick slow yoga routine with a focus on postures that relax your abdominal region. When you're done eating, put on an oversized blanket, drink the warm water infused with lemon honey before taking a brief rest. At night, you're surprised by the fact your cramps have drastically decreased.

Once you've begun in a way to align your lifestyle and diet to the wisdom of Ayurveda particularly when you are going through menstrual cycles, it's more than managing symptoms; it's an opportunity to take care of yourself and a deeper understanding of your body.

ADDRESSING COMMON ISSUES: PMS, IRREGULARITIES, AND MORE

In the case of many women, the period leading up to menstrual cycle can be just as difficult and, in some cases, more difficult as the actual menstrual cycle itself. The pre-menstrual disorder (PMS) can be characterized as an array of emotions and physical symptoms as well as other irregularities in menstrual flow, affect women's lifestyle. Ayurveda offers a way to comprehend these problems and suggests practical strategies for addressing these issues.

PMS: MORE THAN JUST MOOD SWINGS

The term PMS can be interpreted as it being "moody" or "sensitive" However, for women who are experiencing the condition, it's a lot more. It can be a sign of swelling and tenderness in the breasts to mood disorders and irritability.

Dietary adjustments: To stop bloating, decrease the amount of salt you consume. Incorporate magnesium-rich food items like greens and nuts to ease mood fluctuations. Additionally, cut down on caffeine and sugar intake, as they can cause the symptoms of mood disorders and cause breast tenderness.

The herbal allies Chaste Tree berry as well as evening primrose oil are well-known for their capability to ease PMS symptoms. Similar to that, Ayurvedic herbs like Shatavari help balance hormones of females and provide relief.

Reduce Stress: Because stress can trigger symptoms of PMS taking a step towards reducing stress including meditation or slow walks can prove advantageous.

MENSTRUAL IRREGULARITIES: BRINGING BALANCE BACK

Periods that are irregular can indicate deeper imbalances. Although it is important to talk with your doctor, Ayurveda offers supplementary guidance.

Regulate Digestion: According to Ayurveda an optimum digestive system is a cornerstone for general health. Incorporate digestive spices such as turmeric, ginger as well as fennel into your food items. Regular eating habits may also aid in providing the menstrual cycle into a regular rhythm.

Exercise regularly Exercise moderately to increase blood flow and assist in controlling the flow of your menstrual cycle.

Ayurvedic treatments: Basti or Ayurvedic enema with specific oils, or herbal decoctions can aid in some cases. Always seek advice from an Ayurvedic doctor prior to undergoing any treatment procedure.

Treatment of Other Problems: Menorrhagia (heavy bleeding) or Dysmenorrhea (painful menstrual cycles) are two issues women are faced with. Utilizing cold compresses and aloe vera gel may ease the heavy flow. Warm compresses containing lavender oil or chamomile help ease suffering.

A Practical Example: Meet Tara. Each month, as if by it was clockwork Tara was feeling irritable, full of gas, as well as suffering from a throbbing headache it was a sure indicator of her coming menstrual cycle. Following a recommendation from a close friend, Tara decided to try the Ayurvedic method. She started drinking the teas of ginger and fennel throughout the day. It did not just improve her digestion however it significantly decreased bloating. Incorporating magnesium-rich foods such as spinach and almonds helped reduce the mood fluctuations. Also, she made time each morning to do deep breathing exercises that made her feel more calm and relaxed.

In Ayurveda female health issues aren't isolated issues and are a reflection of the total health of the body.

EMPOWERING PRACTICES FOR EMOTIONAL WELL-BEING

Menstrual cycles aren't only an experience in the physical sense, it is deeply connected to our mental landscape. When hormones fluctuate and change emotions may ride an up and down that leaves many feeling completely stressed or out of their element. Ayurveda recognizes the intricate relationship between mind and body and provides methods to assist women to achieve emotional equilibrium and tranquility.

THE POWER OF SELF-AWARENESS

Before tackling remedies It is essential to comprehend the value of self-awareness. When one is aware of their emotional state and being aware of patterns and patterns, you can detect and handle emotional changes throughout menstrual cycles. A simple journal of mood is a great way to gain insight by revealing triggers and the patterns that can cause emotional stress.

MIND-NOURISHING FOODS

Diet is a key factor for emotional well-being. Certain foods may trigger emotions, while other foods are able to soothe and calm. Incorporating grounding food items like roots vegetables, nutritious Ghee and warm prepared meals may have an euphoric effect on your mind. The flipside is that the reduction of stimulants like caffeine or refined sugars may help prevent depression.

DAILY RITUALS FOR BALANCE

Ayurveda highlights the importance regular routines for maintaining the emotional health of people:

Abhyanga (Self-massage) using warm coconut oil or sesame A daily massage can help calm the nervous system, and give an overall sense of groundedness and self-love.

Meditation: Just an hour of concentrated breath or guided meditation may help you create a calm and peaceful space that acts as a stabilizing force when times are turbulent.

EMBRACING NATURE

The act of spending time outdoors in any way, be it a tranquil stroll in the park, as well as listening to sounds of the waves, can provide an effect of grounding. Nature is a reminder of our cycles, and provides perspectives and peace.

SEEKING COMMUNITY AND SUPPORT

The sharing of experiences and feelings in a safe group of friends or group can be a great way to heal. Sometimes, the simple fact that you're not the only one with similar experience can make all the world of distinction.

An actual example: Anika always dreaded her menstrual cycles, not due to physical discomfort, rather due to the emotional stress the experience brought. After one particularly difficult month, she sought out Ayurveda for help. Then she started to incorporate the warm and grounding food items into her daily diet. She also began an evening routine that included massages by herself followed by minutes of relaxation. The practices, along and monthly meetings of a women's group support changed her experience of menstrual flow. Instead of fearing menstrual cramps, she viewed menstrual periods as an opportunity to engage in reflection and self-care.

Affirming your emotional health is just as important as dealing with physical ailments. When you understand the particular issues that the menstrual cycle offers and by implementing Ayurvedic methods, women are able to manage this period with ease and confidence.

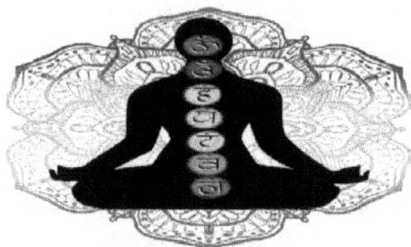

Chapter 3: Ayurvedic Pregnancy And Postpartum Care

PREPARING THE BODY FOR PREGNANCY

The process of pregnancy, as described in Ayurveda is considered to be an experience that is profoundly transformative and not only for the body but for the spirit. Because it's the container to birth a new baby it is vital that the body is at its best health. Let's look at the way Ayurveda recommends preparing your body to embark on this journey of a lifetime:

BALANCING DOSHAS

Prior to conception, it is essential to maintain the balance of three doshas: Vata, Pitta, and Kapha. A mismatch can impact fertility as well as the general wellbeing of the baby. An energizing diet that is specific to your type of dosha along with appropriate habits of living, will help attain this balance.

DETOXIFYING THE SYSTEM

The notion of detoxifying also known as Shodhana is a key concept in Ayurveda. In the beginning it's important to clean the body of any toxins that may have been accumulated. This is accomplished by panchakarma therapies under the supervision by an Ayurvedic practitioner. A simple home detox could involve drinking warm water, including food items that cleanse, and staying away from foods that are processed or contaminated.

NOURISHING DIET

The process of building Ojas (vital vital energy) is essential to fertility. The foods rich in life-giving energy - like dates, ghee and almonds as well as whole grains are recommended. Drinking regularly a beverage made of milk, which is sweetened by honey or dates, and with the addition of a little cardamom is also beneficial.

EMOTIONAL AND MENTAL WELLNESS

An unflinching mind and positive emotional state play an important part in the conception process. Stress is a major issue for couples attempting to have a baby. Strategies like yoga, meditation, and deep breathing exercises may help you relax and promote an attitude of positivity.

REGULARIZING THE MENSTRUAL CYCLE

Menstrual cycles that are regular and consistent can be a reliable indication of the health of your reproductive system. If you are experiencing irregularity, Ayurveda recommends herbs like Shatavari as well as Ashwagandha. Always consult an Ayurvedic expert before taking any herb.

STRENGTHENING PHYSICAL HEALTH

Simple exercises, yoga poses specially designed to promote the fertility (like yoga poses like Baddha Konasana or Butterfly Pose) along with regular strolls can improve your physical health and endurance. They can also prepare your body for the demands of a pregnancy.

DEEPENING CONNECTION WITH PARTNER

The process of conception is not only an act of physical birth, but rather it is a union between two souls. Spending time together and communicating, understanding each the other's expectations and anxieties regarding parenthood and cultivating the bond of physical and emotional bond can help during the birth process.

An example: Rhea and Vikram were looking forward to starting their own family. But after a couple of months of perseverance the traditional methods, they chose to go with the Ayurvedic strategy. Rhea began a slow cleanse, altered her diet to include healthier foods and started daily meditation. Vikram also joined in the practices. After a couple of months, not only did they both feel better physically as well, but they were also more connected emotionally to each other as couples. After a while the couple was thrilled to learn that the couple was expecting.

NOURISHING THE MOTHER-TO-BE: DIET AND ROUTINES

The time of pregnancy is an incredibly important phase of a woman's existence in which she nurtures an embryo within her, as well as undergoes a profound change her. Ayurveda insists on taking care of both body and body during this time. The health of the mother directly influences the development and health of the infant. This is how Ayurveda suggests feeding the mother-to-be:

WHOLESOME DIET

It's the time to enjoy dishes which can be described as Sattvic in nature. That is to say, they're pure, vital and natural. They are vital, essential, and filled with life. Mother-to-bes should be focused on:

Fresh fruit and vegetables are a great source of vitamins as well as minerals. In particular, leaves of greens provide iron as well as folic acid. Both are essential for the development of babies.

Whole grain: Diets such as wheat, rice, and oats are high in the fiber as well as energy.

Dairy: Ghee, milk butter, and milk do not only supply calcium, they additionally enhance the Ojas by boosting health and resilience.

Proteins Lentils Pulses, lentils as well as in certain diets, the consumption of lean meats is advantageous. They meet the demands of the infant and mother's body.

HYDRATION

drinking enough water is essential. Beyond that, drinking the herbal teas that contain ginger, peppermint or Chamomile may help digestion as well as offer a relaxing experience. Fruit juices that are fresh and free of artificial sugars, may provide a nutritious alternative.

ROUTINE AND REST

Regularity in your daily routine can help to ground the new mother. It includes regular meal times as well as sleep schedules as well as relaxation routines. A good night's rest is essential. An hour of rest in the afternoon is a great way to refresh the body.

MINDFUL MOVEMENT

While vigorous activities aren't advised, moderate exercises as well as prenatal yoga are extremely helpful. They improve circulation, ease discomfort and also aid in preparing the body for childbirth.

SELF-CARE RITUALS

Self-massage, also known as Abhyanga, using warm sesame oil or specific medicated oil is very nourishing. It does not only provide moisture to the skin, it also gives relief and may even help prevent stretch marks. After the massage, an ice bath will increase the benefits.

MENTAL AND EMOTIONAL CARE

The pleasure of reading uplifting novels, listening to relaxing music or participating in creative pursuits is a great way to feel satiated. Beware of stressful or overly stimulating areas is also suggested.

An example: Meera, an expectant mother, developed an annual ritual to begin the day with a cup of warm milk, topped with a little honey and turmeric. This did not just provide her the calcium she needed, but it was also a way to start the day on a calm note. Following that, a brief stroll around the yard, taking in the sounds of birds and setting a serene tone throughout the remainder of the day. At weekends she'd take part in a self-massage that was her favorite self-care routine.

POSTPARTUM   RECOVERY   AND
REJUVENATION

The postpartum period, commonly called"the "fourth trimester", is an extremely delicate time. Although the excitement of welcoming an infant to the world is unbeatable but the mind and body of a newly-born mother go through major transformations. It is a crucial time to heal, building strength as well as bonding with the baby. Ayurveda is a holistic treatment for postpartum to ensure that the newborn mom feels rejuvenated and supported.

DEEP NOURISHMENT

The body post-childbirth is under immense stress and is depleted of vital fluids. It's vital to replenish it by:

Warm, cooked and digestible food. Porridges, soups, broths and stews are nutritious and comforting.

Include ghee into your diet as it's thought to help lubricate organs in the body as well as aid in the healing process.

Foods high in protein and iron, such as lentils and green leafy vegetables, and meats that are lean are a great way to recover from muscle and blood loss as well as repair.

HERBAL ASSISTANCE

Certain Ayurvedic herbal remedies can prove invaluable in this time:

Shatavari is considered to be a blessing for women. It balances hormones, boosts lactation and improves overall health.

Ashwagandha is a great remedy for depression and postpartum fatigue.

The combination of saffron and turmeric warm milk are able to provide soothing as well as a boost in mood.

REST AND SLEEP

Do not underestimate the importance of sleep. Although caring for a new baby may disrupt regular sleep patterns Achieving a restful night every time possible is crucial. A well-rested mom is able to care for her infant more effectively.

GENTLE MOVEMENTS

While it's crucial to be restful however, it's equally crucial to slowly reintroduce activity. Light walks, yoga after birth or simple stretches are a great way to improve circulation, increase spirits, and help in speedier recovery.

WARM OIL MASSAGES

Massage the body using warm oils is beneficial for strengthening muscles, relieving joint pain, and bringing relief. It is a soothing practice that can also assist in battling postpartum depression.

EMOTIONAL SUPPORT

The new mom goes through an array of emotions. It's crucial to have a solid emotional support network, whether that's friends, family or a professional. The sharing of feelings, worries as well as joys and worries can be very beneficial.

An example: Priya, after her birth, was overwhelmed by a sense of excitement and a sense of exhaustion. The mother of her child introduced her to the ancient ritual of receiving a warm oil massage, followed by the bathing in water that was that was infused with herbs for healing. The ritual not only soothed her body, but it also offered the perfect space to be in touch with her. Her husband ensured that she had a cup of tea with herbal ingredients at her side at night, making sure that she was well-hydrated and relaxed.

The postpartum process isn't only focused on healing the body. it's about nurturing the spirit and ensuring that mother is appreciated, loved and well-taken care of. The Ayurvedic approach is holistic looking at the newborn mother as a source of affection and vitality, who deserves absolute care.

BALANCING MENTAL HEALTH AFTER BIRTH

A new baby is an incredibly emotional experience that changes not just the body of a woman, but also her thoughts. The complicated hormonal dance, along with the enormous obligation and new routines frequently cause emotions that are tense. The Ayurvedic approach can be an empathetic role in maintaining the mental health of newborns.

RECOGNIZING THE CHANGES

It's crucial to recognize that experiencing the whirlwind of emotions typical. From joy to exhaustion, from excitement to anxiety and more, all of it is element of our journey. Ayurveda is a firm believer in acknowledging the feelings and honoring them and not ignoring these feelings.

NURTURING WITH NUTRITION

The well-balanced and balanced diet plays an important role in stabilizing mood shifts.

Nuts or flaxseeds as well as fatty fish that are rich in Omega-3s are believed as a way to treat depression.

Incorporating entire grains and fresh fruit and veggies can provide the steady flow of energy that keeps the mood swings in check.

Herbal teas, such as the chamomile and tulsi teas, may help to relax.

MEDITATION AND MINDFULNESS

If it's only for a short time it can give you calm and a sense of clarity. It assists in grounding a mommy, and permits her to reconnect to her own inner being amidst the chaotic.

An example: Ayesha, with her second child, was incredibly stressed. Five minutes of concentrated breathing each day helped her feel a the feeling of calm and peace.

HERBAL ALLIES

Herbs such as Shankhpushpi as well as Brahmi are revered in Ayurveda for their calming properties. It is possible to consume them in conjunction to an Ayurvedic practitioner to promote your mental health and decrease anxiety.

SELF-CARE RITUALS

It's vital for any new mom to make time for some "me-time". This isn't about selfishness, but self-preservation. It doesn't matter if you're reading a book or taking a bath, savoring music, or just relaxing with an face mask, these simple practices can help to rejuvenate your mind.

TALK THERAPY

Talking can heal. Talking about your feelings, worries anxieties, worries, and pleasures with a confidant who is trusted, regardless of whether they are a partner or a family member, friend or even a professional, could be a therapeutic experience.

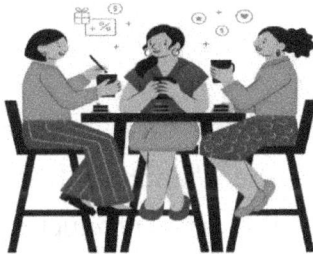

Chapter 4: Navigating Menopause With Grace

WHAT AYURVEDA SAYS ABOUT MENOPAUSE

Menopausal symptoms, commonly referred to as the 'change of life', is actually a normal and necessary period in women's lives. Instead of seeing it as the end of the world, Ayurveda sees it as an opportunity to begin anew, as the beginning of the next phase of your life. It is something that should be taken by a sense of calm and wisdom. We'll explore the way the ancient holistic system views menopausal changes.

THE THREE STAGES OF LIFE

In Ayurveda the life cycle is split into three major stagesthe "Kapha' (the stage of growth)and Pitta (the productive stage) as well as Vata (the stage of wisdom, or the stage of enlightenment). Menopausal transitions signify the change from the Pitta phase, which is often linked with productivity and midlife and productivity, to the Vata phase where women enter their age of wisdom.

NATURAL, NOT A DISEASE

In contrast to some contemporary views that refer to menopausal as a medical problem, Ayurveda regards it as a natural process. Menopausal symptoms occur when the energy of a woman's reproductive system is preserved and directed towards enhancing her understanding as well as spirituality and knowledge.

THE INFLUENCE OF DOSHAS

The signs and symptoms of menopausal symptoms vary between women, and Ayurveda is adamant that this can be attributed to one's dominant dosha. A Pitta-dominant woman could have more frequent hot flashes as compared to women with a Vata woman might be more troubled with insomnia or anxiety.

BALANCING THE ELEMENTS

Menopausal symptoms are a sign that the element of fire (associated to Pitta) is diminished, while the elements of space and air (linked in Vata) take over. This can cause various emotional and physical changes. Ayurveda can provide suggestions on how to balance these elements shifts to help ensure a more smooth change.

EMBRACING THE WISDOM YEARS

The Vata stage, the menopausal phase introduces, is typically linked to profound insight that are heightened in the sense of intuition and spiritual growth. Women are encouraged to take advantage of these talents, channeling their efforts into endeavors which nourish their souls as well as benefit the community.

NATURAL REMEDIES FOR MENOPAUSAL SYMPTOMS

Menopausal symptoms can be a myriad of symptoms, from hot flashes and evening sweats, to mood swings and insomnia. Even though these changes may be difficult, Ayurveda provides an array of remedies that are natural for easing the transition making sure women go through the transition with minimal pain and with maximum pleasure. Let's take a look at mild and powerful Ayurvedic strategies for managing the symptoms of menopausal.

1. HERBAL ALLIES

Ashwagandha is an anti-aging herb, Ashwagandha is excellent for relaxing the nervous system as well as decreasing anxiety. It can also help you sleep more soundly which is something that many women want when they enter menopausal.

Shatavari The herb often called"the "queen of herbs" for women. It's helpful for the symptoms of hot flashes, mood swings and hormone balance, helping to soothe and cool internal organs of the body.

Black Cohosh: A popular herbal remedy for supporting menopausal women, Black Cohosh can alleviate the symptoms of night sweats, mood disorders, as well as hot flashes.

2. DIET ADJUSTMENTS

A diet that is Vata-pacifying could be especially beneficial in menopausal. You should choose moist, warm and grounding food items in preference to dry, cold foods. Consider nourishing soups, steaming veggies, and hearty grain. Ghee (clarified butter) is also beneficial because of its nurturing and lubricating qualities.

3. DAILY ROUTINES FOR BALANCE

Making a habit can be very stabilizing. This could be:

Self-massage (Abhyanga) Warm sesame oil is deeply nourishing, aiding in the healing of the dry, flaky skin that is one of the main complaints of menopausal women.

Daily meditation routine, even for a short time, will help to calm the mind, and help manage emotions.

Gentle Yoga: Positions such as forward bends or child's posture can be relaxing, and tree poses can assist to balance and strengthen your grounding.

4. COOLING PRACTICES

If you're who are struggling with hot flashes:

Moon Bathing: Spending your time in the cool glow of the moon is cool and refreshing.

Sipping cool water Infuse your drinks with cucumber mint, rose petals for a refreshing impact.

5. EMOTIONAL AND SPIRITUAL CARE

The menopausal cycle isn't just an emotional and physical change, but it is as well an emotional and spiritual one. Writing, taking time to be outdoors, participating in women's clubs or getting counseling help on this higher scale.

Be aware that every woman's experience of menopausal symptoms is different for each woman. It's important to listen to your body and be in touch with your body and adapt your treatments according to your needs. Most importantly, you should take advantage of this as a time to explore your own self and for profound development. The menopausal experience, despite its difficulties is also an incredibly enriching process particularly when it is accompanied by knowledge from Ayurveda.

LIFESTYLE ADJUSTMENTS FOR VITALITY

When women enter menopausal, some modifications in their lives could make all the changes, helping them maintain vitality, happiness and vitality. Based on Ayurveda the menopausal phase is perceived as not a medical issue however, as an natural stage of life. With the proper life choices, this period is as exciting and rewarding as the other. Below are some ways to adjust your day-to-day routine so that you maintain your vitality:

Establishing the rhythm Your body is a natural rhythm. You should wake up and fall asleep around the same time every day. If our body is aware of what it is expected to do and when to expect it, it manages better with energy.

Keep active: Although intense exercises may not be the best choice however, there are plenty of ways to remain active. Think about activities such as swimming, walking or even gentle yoga, which provide an exercise that is not too strenuous on the body.

Eat mindfully: Enjoy meals free of distractions. Consume food at intervals that maintain blood sugar levels. Focus on foods that are healthy as well as whole and easy to absorb. Menopausal symptoms can affect the digestion process, and therefore paying attention to the body's signals is crucial.

Be Hydrated: During hormonal fluctuations, your demands for water in the body can change. Make sure you drink lots of fluids throughout your entire all day. Herbal teas, particularly ones with cooling herbs may also prove beneficial.

Beware of Overstimulation: During this stage, it's very easy to get overwhelmed or stressed. Reduce the amount of screen time you spend in the evening, particularly prior to bedtime, and make an effort to participate with calming pursuits like the reading of a book or listening to relaxing music.

Engage in creative Pursuits: Menopause often brings the feeling of having a fresh confidence in yourself and a sense of creativity. Engage in activities that you enjoy whether it's gardening, painting, writing and even dancing. Being expressive can improve your the mood and boost your energy levels.

Connect with friends: spend time with your beloved ones. Engaging in conversations that are meaningful while laughing, sharing stories and stories can bring you back to yourself.

Be sure to take care of yourself: Don't underestimate the value of a soothing bath, reading a good book or relaxing day at the spa. Self-care moments can revitalize you and make your feel happier and energetic.

Stop taking stimulants: Limit your intake of alcohol, caffeine as well as sugar. These are known to trigger hot flashes and impact the quality of sleep. Focus instead on healthy and nutritious meals.

Look for Balance: Always remember that it's fine to let go. If you're struggling to stay sane take care to prioritize your wellbeing over the demands of your job. You can relax and replenish.

An example: Mira, a 52-year-old teacher, began her menopausal experience feeling exhausted and stressed. Making small adjustments, such as walking every day, doing meditation and taking an art class her experience was feeling more positive and happy as she's been in many years. The changes she made that were influenced by Ayurvedic concepts, changed her experience of menopausal change from being a struggle into empowering.

EMOTIONAL AND SPIRITUAL GUIDANCE

Menopausal acceptance isn't just dealing with physical changes, but it is also about nourishing the spiritual and emotional dimensions of a person's life. Ayurveda recognizes that the process of going through menopausal transitions is deeply connected with the woman's emotional as well as spiritual development. Menopausal time, also known in the context of being"the "second spring" in a woman's existence, could be an occasion for self-reflection discovery, self-discovery, as well as profound development.

Becoming a Change-maker: Know menopausal symptoms are a natural process that is not a condition. This is a time when women gain greater understanding of herself. Making the decision to accept this change instead of avoiding it, could create a more calming emotional terrain.

The process of gaining self-awareness is often a mirror reflection of unresolved problems or anger that is suppressed. This is a great moment to reflect on your own. The practice of journaling or meditation may provide insight into the inner life of one by revealing habits or ideas which require more attention.

Finding Support: Speaking to anyone - whether it's an experienced friend, someone from the family, or even a therapist may provide comfort. Talking about your experiences will bring relief and clarity. You might consider joining support groups in which women talk about their experiences as menopausal providing information and support.

Developing Gratitude: focusing on blessings while establishing the habit of gratitude could shift your perspective. Through recognizing and appreciating the world's blessings - whether small or large it can help to develop an optimistic mindset as well as mental resilience.

Connecting to Nature: Take some time outside. Nature is therapeutic that provides solace and a sense of grounded. If it's taking a stroll through the parks taking care of a garden or relaxing by the stream being in nature could provide a deep rejuvinating experience for your soul.

Engaging in Spirituality: For a lot of it is the time to open up towards a deeper spiritual relationship. Find religious practices that appeal to you. This could be prayer and attending religious gatherings or even reading inspirational books.

Engage with Creative Expression: Channel emotions into creative expression. Dance, write, paint or even sing. These creative outlets are beneficial, allowing you to deal with and express emotions.

Try Mindfulness-based and Meditation These methods can aid in managing mood swings as well as provide an atmosphere of peace. Just a short amount of time spent in focused meditation or breathing can help to calm the mind, and offer the emotional stability.

Chapter 5: Unveiling Your Dosha

DISCOVERING YOUR UNIQUE BODY TYPE

Ayurveda the oldest practice of living is a constant reminder that everyone is special. It's not just an expression of poetry and is founded in a physical and mental system that controls how we respond to our surroundings. This is the framework Ayurveda describes as a person's "dosha" or body type. It is similar to having a personal guideline to your optimal wellbeing.

THE ESSENCE OF DOSHAS:

In Ayurveda the universe as well as all that is within it, even our own bodies, are composed of five elements that are fundamental that include space (ether) air as well as water, fire and earth. Combining these elements makes up the three main doshas: Vata, Pitta, and Kapha. Each individual is a distinct mixture of these doshas which determines their physical traits as well as their mental capabilities, mental tendencies and their vulnerability to specific diseases.

WHY IT MATTERS:

Imagine you could have an outline of your own. The knowledge of your predominant dosha can give you this. It helps you make the right choices for your diet as well as suggests the best exercise routines as well as aids in managing stress and also assists to build more harmonious relations. In essence, knowing the dosha of your body helps to live in harmony with the natural world around you.

DETERMINING YOUR DOSHA:

Although one could seek expert consulting to establish their primary dosha, there are a few self-assessment tools also. Examining the physical characteristics, such as the body's frame as well as skin type and hair type, in conjunction with observing one's personal emotions, preferences, and sleep pattern could provide indications. There are many Ayurvedic websites also provide questions that help people identify their dosha.

FINE-TUNING YOUR OBSERVATIONS:

Although self-assessment may give you some general information however, it's important to recognize that the vast majority of us are some combination of doshas which means that one is more dominant than others. There is also the possibility for a dosha balances to change because of various reasons like the environment, age and tension. Thus, regular assessments can be useful.

An example: Maya, always a strong and agile woman experienced anxiety and suffering from insomnia. Although she initially attributed it to workplace stress, a visit with an Ayurvedic practitioner revealed an increased Vata within her body. Confronting her Vata dominance as well as the present imbalance, she was provided with tailored suggestions for lifestyle, diet and techniques for relaxation. As time passed, and with regular use, she noticed an improvement in overall health and health.

In a time when one-size-fits-all solutions are commonly offered Ayurveda's focus on individuality is like a breath fresh air. When you discover and understand your individual body's characteristics it allows you to choose choices that are in alignment with your natural nature, helping to promote health, vitality and peace in your life.

TAILORED DIETARY GUIDELINES

Each bite consumed is not simply nutrition, but the message we transmit the body. According to Ayurveda knowing the dosha of a person is crucial since it is a key factor in determining which foods affect or upset your body's balance. We'll explore the ways in which Ayurveda formulates diet recommendations in accordance with your dosha.

VATA - THE WIND ENERGY:

If you're mostly Vata (associated with the elements of air and space) the body and brain are naturally fast as well as light and cool. There's a possibility that you'll be inclined toward dry skin, fast thoughts, or perhaps some restlessness. The digestive system can appear inconsistent.

Foods to Eat Hot warm, cooked, and moist meals such as stews, soups, and stews. The root vegetables, grains such as wheat and rice dairy, nut products as well as seeds can be healthy.

Things to avoid: Raw, cold and dry food items. Consumption of too many beverages, cold salads or excessive caffeine may increase Vata.

For morning breakfast Sarah who is Vata kind of person, prefers an oatmeal bowl warm that is topped with stewed apples, cinnamon and a touch of ghee in place of her usual choice chilled smoothie.

PITTA - THE FIRE ENERGY:

If you're predominantly Pitta (associated with water and fire elements) You radiate warmth, possess a strong digestion and may have a fiery temperament. Skin conditions could be very sensitive or susceptible to rashes.

What To Eat: Cold dry, somewhat dry and hefty foods. Consider salads, dairy grains, such as barley and rice, and protein sources like turkey and chicken.

Avoid Oily, hot, spicy or fermented food because they can cause more harm to your Pitta fire.

An example: Rohan, with his Pitta constitution, discovered the switch of spicy curries to grilled chicken salads, not only slowed his heartburn, but also helped him feel more energetic.

KAPHA - THE EARTH ENERGY:

If you're predominantly Kapha (related to earth elements and water) You're naturally serene, stable, and sturdy. There is a tendency toward weight gain and slowness.

What To Eat: Light warming, hot and spicy food items. Choose vegetables such as spinach and broccoli, as well as grains like millet and barley and other spices, such as black pepper and ginger.

Avoid Oily, heavy, or cold meals. In excess of dairy products such as fried or fried foods and sweets could cause Kapha unsteady.

An example: Maria, a Kapha type, was once a fan of her pasta with a cheesy flavor, but later changed to stir-fries made of vegetables and the addition of quinoa. It didn't only aid in losing weight but also added more energy in her day-to-day activities.

In Ayurveda it is believed that food serves as the primary source of treatment. If we select foods that match with the dosha of our constitution, we're not only giving our body food, we're providing nourishment to our souls as well as ensuring that all cellular functions function perfectly. If the food choices are compatible with the body's constitution and constitution, it results in not only physical health but mental stability and clarity.

PERSONALIZED BEAUTY AND SELF-CARE ROUTINES

Ayurveda commonly referred to by its name as the "science of life", is a holistic method that doesn't just focus on the internal state of health, but encompasses our outer appearance and how we treat our body. It is based on the idea that beauty comes out of an internal harmony, Ayurveda offers insights into specific self-care and beauty routines that are based on the dosha of one's. The following are the ways that each dosha will radiate from within:

VATA - THE WIND ENERGY:

For people with a predominantly Vata body, the skin may be rough, dry or cold. Rapid aging is another feature that makes moisture your most valuable asset.

Choose for moisturizing, nourishing products. Massage your skin daily (abhyanga) made with sesame oil is a great way to keep the skin glowing and soft.

For hair care, use conditioning shampoos that hydrate your hair. Massage your scalp regularly using warm sesame or almond oil to fight dryness and dryness.

PITTA - THE FIRE ENERGY:

People with Pitta tend to possess a high body temperature, skin that is sensitive that is prone to irritation, redness or acne. the fine hair can get gray quickly or lose its luster.

Skincare: Use the cooling, soothing, and soft products. Massage with coconut oil can ease the sensitivity. The gel of aloe vera can be an aid to sensitive or red skin.

Haircare: Apply gentle and natural shampoos. Coconut oil is beneficial to massage your scalp, giving cool relief as well as promoting healthy hair.

KAPHA - THE EARTH ENERGY:

The Kapha skin is rich, oily and cool in the hand. The hair is lustrous and wavy. hair. However, they may suffer from problems with their scalp due to oiliness.

Skincare: Gentle, warm and stimulating treatments are the best. You can consider adding an routine of exfoliation to reduce excess oil and to maintain the clarity of your skin.

Haircare: Choose deep cleansing shampoos, and think about including an astringent, such as witch hazel into your scalp maintenance routine.

COMMON SELF-CARE ROUTINES FOR ALL DOSHAS:

Tongue Cleansing: Begin your day with a gentle scrape of your tongue. This Ayurvedic practice helps to eliminate overnight bacterial build-up, and it also helps to stimulate the organs of your internal system.

"Warm Oil Massage Also known as abhyanga, the full body warm oil massage is nourishing for the skin and aids in lymphatic drainage and provides a feeling of being grounded.

Eye care Washing your eyes frequently by using cool, refreshing water or drops of rose water for eyes will keep them looking fresh and healthy.

Meditation Practices: Everyday practice of meditation, even if only for a short amount of time will help keep your mental wellbeing in balance and enhance your overall health.

If it's Vata, Pitta, or Kapha Understanding the doshas that you have and adjusting your self-care and beauty routines helps you to achieve your internal balance, revealing the genuine beauty. As Ayurveda says, beauty encompasses your body, mind as well as the soul.

EMOTIONAL BALANCE FOR EACH DOSHA

Ayurveda is a system of medicine that, thanks to its sensitive understanding of the human condition is aware that our feelings aren't a separate thing. They're closely linked to our health, the environment, and specifically the dosha type we have. In recognizing and analyzing the patterns of emotion that be triggered by each dosha you can more effectively navigate through the turmoil of our emotions which will bring greater peace and peace. This is how each dosha can be associated with specific emotions and the best way to align these:

VATA - THE WIND ENERGY:

Vatas due to their refreshing and light-hearted characteristics, are usually imaginative, energetic, and lively. If they are imbalanced, they could feel anxious and restlessness. or even a sense of sluggishness.

Balancing tips: Grounding exercises like walking with bare feet on grass or in the dirt and consistent habits, warming and nutritious foods, as well as deeply breathing exercises may help bring peace. The practice of meditation, particularly targeted or guided practices could provide the mental support Vata people sometimes require.

PITTA - THE FIRE ENERGY:

Pittas who are fuelled by the elements of water and fire they are driven, passionate and keen-minded. But, if their passion is not controlled, it may be manifested as anger, frustration anger, jealousy, or a lot of criticism.

Balance Tips Relaxing and cooling activities like evening walks, swimming or just being in the water, may help. Food wise, try to avoid sweet or acidic meals which can stoke internal fires. Engaging in compassion-based (also known as loving kindness (Metta) meditation could aid in calming the fire-breathing Pitta nature.

Chapter 6: Integrating Ayurveda With Modern Medicine

THE SCIENCE BEHIND AYURVEDIC REMEDIES

Ayurveda is often described as the "science of life," has been around for a long the years, offering holistic healing over hundreds of years. Although modern medicine primarily revolves around the treatment of symptoms, Ayurveda delves deep into the root of the issue, and addresses all aspects of a person's life: body, mind and soul.

A GLIMPSE INTO AYURVEDIC PHARMACOLOGY:

In Ayurveda each herb, plant or mineral can be considered medicinal and is often utilized in complex mixtures to produce balanced formulations. They are not just designed to ease symptoms, but also to restore harmony in the doshas of your body. In the case of turmeric, for instance, the gold spice turmeric, now worldwide acclaimed is rooted in Ayurveda. Curcumin is an active ingredient that is found in turmeric, is acknowledged for its powerful anti-inflammatory and antioxidant qualities.

EVIDENCE-BASED AYURVEDA:

Since the last decade The intersection between Ayurveda as well as scientific research has grown. Many research studies have been carried out to verify the efficacy of Ayurvedic treatments.

Ashwagandha known as an adaptogen has been researched to determine its effectiveness in relieving anxiety and stress. The latest research confirms the fact that it has the ability to decrease cortisol levels which are the primary stress hormone in our body.

Triphala the traditional mix comprised of three different fruits has been recognized as a powerful ingredient in promoting the digestion process and maintaining regular stool movement. New research has shown its positive effects on gut bacteria and its role to improve the health of your colon.

Brahmi (Bacopa monnieri) is revered as a herb that helps improve mental clarity and mind-set in Ayurveda. Recent research has confirmed the benefits of its neuroprotective effects and also for improving cognitive abilities.

COMPLEMENTARY APPROACHES:

Modern medicine's strength lies in precise diagnosis, emergency treatment as well as surgical techniques for taking care of acute ailments. Ayurveda excels in the field of preventive medicine and chronic disease management and overall wellbeing development. If they are used in conjunction it can offer an all-encompassing strategy for well-being. As an example although modern medicine could provide oral hypoglycemics or insulin for managing diabetes Ayurveda is able to complement this by recommending lifestyle and diet adjustments to correct the root issues that cause the problem. The scientific basis of Ayurvedic treatments isn't only found in old texts, it's constantly confirmed by the latest studies. Integrating both Ayurveda and modern science is a holistic method of combining ancient wisdom with modern research to promote maximum health and wellness. However, it's important to seek out medical professionals prior to switching between therapies to make sure that the treatment is safe and effective.

POTENTIAL INTERACTIONS AND PRECAUTIONS

In the current era of fusion of Ayurveda alongside modern medicine It is essential to proceed cautiously. Similar to all other medicines, Ayurvedic remedies, while naturally derived, could interfere with other medicines, which can have unexpected effects. Understanding these possible interactions will ensure that we get benefits from both without risking our health.

AYURVEDIC REMEDIES AND DRUG INTERACTIONS:

Each remedy, whether it's an herbal remedy from a pharmacist or a plant from the soil, is infused with the active ingredients that affect our bodies. These effects may enhance, diminish or alter the effects of a different remedy.

Turmeric as well as Blood Thinners The most prominent example is turmeric, which was previously mentioned. Its anti-inflammatory qualities can increase the effectiveness of blood thinners and can lead to increased bleeding.

Ashwagandha and thyroid medication: Ashwagandha, beneficial for its adaptogenic properties, could additionally boost the levels of thyroid hormone. This could be a problem for people who are already taking thyroid medicines, possibly leading to symptoms associated with an overactive thyroid.

Licorice Root as well as Blood Pressure Medicine It is used in Ayurveda for a variety of ailments Licorice can raise blood pressure, thereby reducing the advantages of blood pressure medications.

GAUGING THE DOSAGE:

In Ayurveda it is the dosage that creates the treatment. A dose that is optimal can be effective, whereas an excess dosage can cause side negative effects. Always speak with an Ayurvedic doctor to establish what dosage is appropriate that is appropriate for your particular constitution and situation.

ALLERGIES AND SENSITIVITIES:

The fact that it's natural does not guarantee that it's not prone to side negative effects. There are those who may be sensitized or allergic to particular plants, exhibiting symptoms that range from itching to stomach discomfort.

PURITY OF AYURVEDIC PREPARATIONS:

Make sure that the Ayurvedic products you are taking in are safe and free of pollutants such as heavy metals. When Ayurveda includes treatments that involve the use of metals (known as Bhasmas) These undergo a rigorous process to ensure the safety of. Products that are not regulated may not conform to these guidelines.

PREGNANCY AND LACTATION:

Certain Ayurvedic treatments may not be suitable for pregnant women or during nursing. Some herbs, for instance may stimulate contractions in the uterus or be absorbed into the breast milk.

SEEKING PROFESSIONAL GUIDANCE:

If you are combining Ayurvedic treatments with modern medicine make sure you consult both your doctor and Ayurvedic doctor. They are able to offer insight on possible interactions, and help you choose an appropriate approach to your wellbeing.

FINAL THOUGHTS:

Ayurveda has a wide array of options for a variety of medical issues. However, as with any treatment they come with a range of safeguards. If we are aware, making sure of that we are eating food with the highest quality consume, and seeking professional assistance, we can combine Ayurveda and modern medical practices, resulting in the perfect balance of wellbeing and health.

COMMUNICATING WITH HEALTHCARE PROFESSIONALS

Making the connection between traditional medicine and Ayurveda isn't easy particularly when communicating with health professionals who may not be familiar with Ayurvedic methods. Being open and proactive when you speak to them can make the difference between an unbalanced method and an harmonious combination of the two methods. How can you make sure that your communication is effective:

START WITH TRANSPARENCY:

It's important to talk openly regarding the Ayurvedic treatment or remedies that you're currently undergoing. Do not be shy about it, whether you're undergoing a diet change or a herbal cure or even a particular Ayurvedic treatment you're thinking of.

EDUCATE WITH TACT:

Although some physicians know about Ayurveda and its principles, many may not. If you are confronted with the latter be prepared to approach the issue in a manner that is logical. Offer resources or books on Ayurveda as well as its background and its advantages. Remember, it's never to convince them of your benefits, but instead providing them with a better understanding of your journey to health.

ASK QUESTIONS:

If you're worried about possible interaction or effects that could be harmful Be sure to ask! Examples:

"Do you foresee any problems with taking Ashwagandha alongside my current thyroid medication?"

"I've been doing an Ayurvedic cleanse; how might that impact the blood test you're recommending?"

SCHEDULE REGULAR CHECK-INS:

If you're mixing Ayurvedic as well as conventional therapies is a good idea to get regular checks to keep track of your progress and detect any possible issues in the early stages.

SEEK A MEDIATOR IF NEEDED:

In certain instances you may find it beneficial having your Ayurvedic doctor communicate directly with your physician. They will discuss the specifics of possible interactions and create a the best treatment strategy specifically to you.

UNDERSTAND THE LIMITATIONS:

Although Ayurveda provides an holistic method of healing, traditional medicine can provide specific and urgent care particularly during emergencies. Be aware of the strengths and weaknesses of both, and use both depending on the circumstances.

STAY UPDATED WITH YOUR RECORDS:

A health journal, or a record of your treatments including medications, herbs can prove useful. When you see a health specialist, you will can have the required information in your possession.

ACKNOWLEDGE THE GOAL:

Keep in mind that both your physician as well as your Ayurvedic physician will have your best interests in mind. Through establishing an understanding and mutual respect it is possible to ensure you're getting the most from both possible worlds.

FINAL THOUGHTS:

The principle of open dialogue is at the heart of integrating Ayurveda and the latest medical practices. It allows individuals to manage your health, and to make educated choices, while also ensuring that you're in a secure and efficient path to wellness.

TESTIMONIALS: SUCCESS STORIES OF INTEGRATION

Being able to witness the success of the implementation of Ayurveda alongside modern day medicine could inspire numerous. These testimonials highlight the lives of three people who were able to effortlessly mix the two worlds of Ayurveda and modern medicine and demonstrate the harmony which can be realized by bringing together East is joined by West in the world of health care.

LINDA'S JOURNEY WITH RHEUMATOID ARTHRITIS

For Linda the rheumatoid arthritis condition became a gruelling part of her life. Western medications provided relief however, side effects afflicted her. Linda says "The painkillers numbed my pain, but my body felt alien." After the advent in Ayurveda, Linda began consuming curcumin-based drinks, specifically tailored according to her particular body. In combination with her other conventional medicines, she observed less flare-ups, and an impressive improvement in the pain. "It wasn't just the remedies; it was understanding my body through Ayurveda. My rheumatologist acknowledged the difference, and we worked together to adjust my doses."

RAJ'S BATTLE AGAINST DIABETES

Raj was diagnosed as having Type 2 Diabetes in his late 40s. As insulin and changes in diet kept his blood sugar levels within a certain range, Raj sought a more comprehensive strategy. In the direction by an Ayurvedic physician, Raj was exposed to certain herbs and techniques. "I started incorporating Bitter Melon (Karela) juice and Fenugreek seeds into my diet," Raj says. "I felt more energetic and noticed more stable sugar levels." His endocrinologist was pleased by the results, and over time, assisted Raj to optimize his insulin dose. "It felt like a collaborative effort towards my health, where both systems complemented each other."

SOPHIA'S POSTPARTUM RECOVERY

The birth of Sophia was then followed by depression post-partum. "I felt lost," she recalls. Following the suggestion from a trusted friend, she sought out the services of an Ayurvedic practitioner. As well as her anti-depressants prescribed to her, Sophia began Ayurvedic therapies such as massages, as well as specific diet supplements such as Ashwagandha along with Shatavari. As time passed, she experienced an increasing connection to her child and with herself. "It was as if Ayurveda was filling the gaps, providing not just healing but nourishment to my soul," Sophia explains. Nowadays, Sophia and her gynecologist regularly talk about Ayurvedic knowledge and methods.

These are only an example of the many who've discovered their path to health by taking on both Ayurveda and modern-day medicine. They emphasize the need for reciprocity between both approaches and the importance of the patient as a participant on their journey to health. With more and more people sharing their experiences, they paint an optimistic image of the future in which the pursuit of health is not a decision between different traditions, but rather a integration of the two.

Chapter 7: Ayurvedic Recipes For Radiant Health

BUILDING A BALANCED AYURVEDIC PLATE

With the bustle and craziness of daily life keeping a healthy food regimen is sometimes a distant memory. Yet, Ayurveda emphasizes the importance of our food choices and the way it influences the unique constitution of our body. If you make a healthy Ayurvedic plate it's not just fueling your body, but also providing nourishment to your spirit. Learn how to incorporate traditional wisdom to your contemporary kitchen.

UNDERSTAND THE SIX TASTES (RASAS)

Ayurveda divides food into the six distinct flavors of sweet salted, sour, sharp, bitter and Astringent. An ideal balanced diet will include the flavors of all six and ensures that you are getting many different nutrients. Furthermore, if our taste buds are exposed to all of the flavors mentioned above, it can lead to a greater satisfaction with food and lessens the need for fast food.

THE ROLE OF STAPLES

Rice and wheat: They make up the basis of numerous Ayurvedic food items. As an example, basmati rice is simple to digest and also provides an energy source. If you're looking for something new, explore quinoa and barley. This will ensure that you receive the right amount of amino acids.

PROTEIN SOURCES

Lentils and legumes: Chickpeas, mung beans red lentils, as well as chickpeas are quite popular for Ayurvedic cooking. They are not only full of proteins, but they also contain diet fiber, which is essential for digestion.

VEGETABLES: YOUR DAILY DOSE OF VITAMINS

Local and seasonal vegetables are prominent in Ayurveda. If you consume local food it's not only helping your local community but also obtaining the freshest produce and full of vitality known as "prana".. In the winter season, roots vegetables like beets, carrots, and others are a good choice, and the summer menus can contain bell peppers, zucchinis and other vegetables.

SPICE IT UP!

Spices go beyond flavors enhancers in Ayurveda. Turmeric is known for its anti-inflammatory qualities, and the spice cumin that aids in digestion, are able to be added to food items to offer beneficial benefits for health. It's not just all about making food taste spiced up, but rather harnessing the healing properties of spices.

THE ART OF EATING

The final step in creating a Ayurvedic plate isn't about the food you put on it however, it's also about how you eat it. Savouring every bite and feeling grateful to your food can turn the dining experience into a relaxing one.

PRACTICAL EXAMPLE: A SIMPLE AYURVEDIC MEAL

You can think about lunch plates that include the basmati rice, a lentil soup (dal) with cooked seasonal vegetables that are stir-fried with no spice, and a tiny portion of yogurt as well as a salad that is topped with healthy greens. This dish offers a variety of flavors and textures. You'll are getting a wide range of nutrition.

The way to construct the perfect Ayurvedic plate is similar to painting on a canvas. By combining each component, you can add texture, color and depth. This creates the perfect masterpiece that is nourishing for your body as well as the soul. If you are interested in learning more about Ayurvedic food preparation, you'll experience how satisfying it is to align your diet with nature and your body's requirements and the ancient wisdom which has been promoting wellbeing for thousands of years.

Below are five Ayurvedic recipes to use for your meals:

Breakfast

1. Ayurvedic Porridge:

O Ingredients: Quinoa or Oats, almond milk Ghee and dates, as well as gold raisins, cardamom and Saffron.

Instructions: Cook the Oats or Quinoa within almond milk. When cooked then add a tablespoon of Ghee, chopped dates Golden raisins, and a pinch cardamom and saffron.

2. Warm Cinnamon Apple Cereal:

Ingredients: Sliced apples Cinnamon, cloves Ghee and almond milk.

Instructions: Cook the apples cut into slices in ghee along with one teaspoon each of cloves and cinnamon until they're soft. Serve them with a dash of almond milk.

3. Green Mung Bean Pancakes:

O Ingredients: Soaked green the mung bean, ginger turmeric, cumin seeds rock salt and fresh coriander.

Instructions: Blend the Mung beans that have been soaked into an emulsion. Add finely chopped ginger and the seeds of cumin, turmeric, fresh coriander and salt. Cook pancakes on the grid and serve them with fresh chutney.

4. Spiced Almond Smoothie:

ingredients: Almonds (soaked over night) dates and saffron. Cardamom, saffron as well as cold almond milk.

Instructions Blend the entire mixture until they are smooth. Drink chilled.

5. Sweet Rice & Coconut Breakfast Bowl:

O Ingredients: Basmati rice, coconut milk jaggery (or natural sweetener) as well as cardamom and coconut flakes that have been toasted.

Directions for cooking: cook rice with coconut milk until it becomes tender. Add cardamom and jaggery. Serve with coconut flakes that have been toasted.

Lunch

1. Ayurvedic Kitchari:

The ingredients include: split yellow Mung beans, Basmati Rice and cumin seeds, ghee and turmeric, ginger and a variety of veggies.

Instructions: Saute the spices in ghee. Add rice, mung bean, as well as vegetables. Then add water, and cook until all is cooked.

2. Beetroot & Carrot Stir-Fry:

O ingredients: grated beetroot, carrot, ghee and mustard seeds, curry leaves along with lemon juice.

Instructions to cook: Sauté mustard seeds with Ghee. Then add beetroot, and carrot. Then cook until the vegetables are tender. Finish by adding lemon juice.

3. Spinach and Coconut Curry:

O Ingredients: Spinach Coconut milk, ginger cumin seeds and asafoetida.

Instructions: Cook the spinach in spices till it's they are soft. Mix in coconut milk, and simmer for an additional five minutes.

4. Cooling Cucumber Salad:

Ingredients: Cucumbers that have been chopped yogurt, honey, roast coriander, fresh cumin as well as rock salt.

Instructions: Mix everything with ice then serve it chilled.

5. Ayurvedic Lentil Soup:

The ingredients include red lentils, ghee as well as cumin seeds, ginger and coriander fresh.

Instructions: Cook the lentils until they are soft. Then, cook spices in ghee before mixing with the lentils. Serve with coriander leaves.

Dinner

1. Vegetable Stew:

Other Ingredients: Seasonal vegetables including the coconut milk, cumin seeds as well as curry leaves and ginger.

Instructions: Saute spices in oil for a few minutes, then add the chopped vegetables as well as coconut milk. Let it cook till the vegetables are tender.

2. Turmeric & Ginger Spiced Rice:

The ingredients include: Basmati rice, ghee as well as turmeric, ginger black mustard seeds and lemon juice.

Instructions Cook the rice. Sauté spices in ghee, then blend into the rice. Sprinkle using lemon juice.

3. Mung Bean & Vegetable Soup:

Other Ingredients: Mung Beans along with other veggies Ghee cumin seeds asafoetida, cumin seeds and coriander fresh.

Instructions: Cook Mung beans in vegetable. Cook spices with ghee. mix into the soup. Add fresh coriander.

4. The warm Quinoa Salad with Ghee Roasted Vegetables

O Ingredients: Cooked Quinoa and seasonal vegetables, ghee, lemon juice.

Instructions: Cook vegetables in ghee until golden, then combine with the quinoa. Then, finish with a splash from lemon juice.

5. Fennel & Mint Digestive Tea (to drink post-dinner):

O Ingredients Include: Fennel seeds, fresh mint leaves, as well as honey.

Instructions: Boil the mint leaves and fennel seeds. Then strain and add honey according to your preference.

The essence of Ayurvedic cooking is using fresh, seasonal and locally available ingredients prepared with passion and love.

REMEDIES FOR COMMON AILMENTS

Ayurveda is a vast experience in the field of spices, herbs and other natural substances, can provide solutions for a wide range of problems with health. In this article, we'll look at several remedies that respond to common illnesses, making sure that you'll be able to find relief through the strength of the natural world.

DIGESTIVE DISCOMFORTS

Lemon Tea and Ginger Lemon Tea: A warm infusion created by infusing fresh ginger slices with lemon juice can aid digestion and ease the feeling of constipation. Ginger increases the digestive fire called 'agni' while lemon functions as an exfoliant.

Cumin-Coriander-Fennel (CCF) Tea: This blend helps in balancing the digestive system. You can boil a teaspoon of the seeds in water. Then strain into a cup, and drink in a relaxing tea.

COLD AND FLU

Tulsi (Holy Basil) Tea: Tulsi is revered in Ayurveda because of its anti-inflammatory qualities. Take a handful of leaves and brew them in hot water, maybe with some honey in order to treat cold symptoms.

Turmeric Milk known as "golden milk," warm milk with a hint of black pepper and turmeric is a soothing treatment for sore throat, and also has anti-inflammatory qualities.

STRESS AND ANXIETY

Ashwagandha commonly referred to as Ayurvedic Ginseng Ashwagandha is known as an adaptogen which can help the body to manage the stress. It is available in tablets or in powder form be sure to consult an Ayurvedic practitioner to determine the appropriate dosage.

Brahmi (Gotu Kola) Tea: This plant is renowned for its relaxing and cognitive-enhancing benefits. A regular intake of the herb can help in decreasing anxiety and improve memory.

SKIN ISSUES

Aloe Vera Gel is great for minor skin irritations or burns The gel of the aloe plant provides cooling relief. It also moisturizes and can be utilized to moisturize your skin naturally.

Neem: Because of its antifungal and antibacterial qualities, neem is beneficial against skin and acne inflammations. Neem leaves are able to be incorporated into a paste that can be put on topically. Neem oil is a good option for cases that are more serious.

SLEEP DISTURBANCES

Chamomile Tea: Although it isn't initially derived taken from Ayurveda, chamomile has been popular due to its relaxing qualities. Warming up with a cup of tea before bed will help you sleep peacefully.

Warm Oil Massage: massaging your soles of your feet using warm sesame oil, or Ghee is a great way to balance your body's energy and help prepare to restful sleeping.

PRACTICAL EXAMPLE: COMBATING FATIGUE

If you're always exhausted or depleted, think about an Ayurvedic tonic that is made up with equal portions honey and the ghee (clarified butter). Consuming a teaspoon every early morning with empty stomachs can help to rejuvenate your body and give you long-lasting energy. The combination of this remedy balances Vata (the Air element that is associated with movements and activity in the nervous system) as well as Pitta (the element of fire that is associated with metabolism and digestion) which results in overall health.

While these solutions are able to provide relief, it's essential to determine the root of every illness. The most severe or chronic symptoms must discuss the issue with a medical specialist. As with all herbal remedy, what performs well for one individual may not work for someone else. So, having a personal awareness and understanding of your body is essential in Ayurveda.

BEAUTY FROM WITHIN: NOURISHING DRINKS AND SNACKS

In Ayurveda aesthetics, beauty on the outside can be a reflection of the inner balance and health. The modern-day beauty rituals usually are focused on the use of topical treatments or cosmetics, Ayurveda emphasizes nourishment from the outside in. When we consume certain beverages and food items that balance doshas, you can get beautiful skin, gorgeous hair, and overall attractive appearance. In this article, we'll explore the various Ayurvedic essentials to promote beautiful appearance from within.

NOURISHING DRINKS:

Golden Turmeric Latte: Turmeric, known for its anti-inflammatory properties, has become an energizing ingredient in Ayurveda. In order to make this drink make a cup of hot milk (cow or almond milk or coconut) mix with half a teaspoon turmeric powder, along with a tiny amount of black pepper (to enhance the intake of curcumin in turmeric) as well as a hint of honey to add the sweetness. This drink is not just good for your immunity, but provides your skin with a healthy glowing appearance.

Rose Petal and Saffron Water A few pieces of saffron as well as some flowers that have dried in a glass of water for a night. The next morning you can strain the water and drink the elixir with an empty stomach. Saffron helps to brighten the skin, while rose cools and calms Pitta dosha. If unbalanced can cause acne and skin irritation.

Amla juice: Amla also known as Indian gooseberry, is a rich source of antioxidants and vitamin C. Consuming it regularly can boost hair growth as well as slow down premature graying. Combine the juice of fresh amlas with water and add some jaggery or honey for sweetness.

NOURISHING SNACKS:

Grilled Makhana (Fox Nuts) The food is lower in calories but packed with nutrients. Protein and calcium are abundant in makhana the makhana supplement hair and skin health.

Then, roast them in a small amount of ghee, and then sprinkle of turmeric and rock salt to make a delicious, healthy snack.

Dates as well as Almond concoction: Dates give an energy and sweetness that is natural, as do almonds, which are loaded with vitamin E which is good for the health of your skin. Incubate 3 to 4 almonds over night and then peel them off in the morning, and then eat along with dates. This easy recipe isn't just delicious, but can also help in rejuvenating the skin cells.

Chickpea flour (Besan) Pancakes Prepare pancake batter using chickpea flour and water and the spices you like (turmeric as well as cumin and coriander). Pan fry the batter to create tasty pancakes. Chickpea flour is rich in protein and is an excellent mineral-rich food source that is essential to maintain skin's elasticity.

PRACTICAL EXAMPLE: ADDRESSING DRY SKIN

If your skin feels tight or dry It could indicate Vata imbalance. Warm drinks to ease Vata is a spicy almond milk. Blend the almonds that have been soaked with warm milk and add the cardamom spice as well as cinnamon and honey. Drinking it regularly, particularly during the colder months will provide a deep-water hydration for the skin. It will give its a firm and youthful appearance.

Beauty is a part of Ayurveda is not just the skin. It's about aligning mind, body and the spirit. This nutritious drink and snack aren't just delicious in taste, but also perform magic on the inside creating the base for natural beauty that sparkles.

DIY AYURVEDIC SKINCARE AND HAIRCARE

Ayurveda, which is a treasure collection of organic ingredients, has a wealth of homemade remedies that can help you ensure the overall well-being of your skin and hair. Let's explore easy but efficient recipes to address the most common hair and skin issues and help you maintain your natural beauty and health.

SKINCARE RITUALS:

Custom-designed face masks for an natural glow blend chickpea meal (besan) and yogurt until you get a smooth paste. Use this mask on your face for about 15 minutes before washing. For acne-prone skin you can add a little turmeric into the mix. To combat dry skin, mix fresh bananas and honey for intense moisture.

Exfoliating Ubtan Combining equal portions of green gram flour and almond powder. Mix in rose water to create a thick paste. Apply the paste gently to your skin with circles, and then cleanse. This traditional recipe cleanses and reenergizes skin.

Rose and Glycerin Toner Combine equal amounts of the rosewater and glycerin. Put it within a spray bottle, and apply it as a refreshing cleanser and setting spray. The product hydrates skin, and also restores the equilibrium in pH.

HAIRCARE SOLUTIONS:

The Nourishing Hair Mask: Mix coconut milk, avocados that are ripe with a teaspoon of honey for the most creamy of masks. Apply it to the root as well as the lengths the lengths of hair. This mask can be a lifesaver for damaged and dry hair. It gives the appearance of softness and shine.

Hibiscus as well as Aloe Vera Gel for hair growth Make a small crush of petals of hibiscus, then mix it in aloe gel. Massage the scalp with it and let it sit for 30 mins before washing. A regular use of this product can help promote hair growth as well as reduce the loss of hair.

Herbal hair rinse: boil leaves of neem along with amla, fenugreek, and seeds in the water. Cool it down and remove the liquid. After shampooing, wash your hair using this herb mix to prevent dandruff. add natural shine to your hair.

PRACTICAL EXAMPLE: COMBATTING HAIR THINNING

If your hair is becoming thinner or falling out too much It could indicate an imbalance of your dosha. typically Pitta. One solution is to massage your scalp using coconut oil that has been infused with some chopped Brahmi leaves. The cooling effects of these ingredients can help to ease Pitta and increase hair follicles to encourage the growth of hair.

Chapter 8: Cultivating A Holistic Lifestyle
THE SIGNIFICANCE OF A DAILY ROUTINE

In today's world of the constant stream of commitments, noise constant notifications making sure you have a solid routine for your day is more important than ever. Ayurveda has always stressed the importance of the importance of a "Dinacharya," or a regular routine that is an essential element for good health long-term health, mental peace. The goal is not to adhere strict to a set schedule however, it's more about creating times of quiet, self-care and self-reflection throughout the day.

WHY IT MATTERS:

Natural Alignment: Our bodies are equipped with an internal clock that syncs with the natural rhythms of nature. When we pay attention to the cycle of the day, such as sunrise noon, sunset, and sunrise We align our energy and activity with natural cycles, maximizing the potential of our bodies.

Consistency can heal: A regular routine is an element of calm. It creates a sense peace, and helps us to stay grounded in all the turmoil. It helps in decreasing anxiety, improving digestion as well as promoting sleep.

Mindfulness and Training: A structured routine helps us be more mindful and present. It could be through morning stretching as well as mindful eating, or even a night of gratitude the daily routines are meditations the moment, creating an inner calm and a sense of focus.

CRAFTING YOUR AYURVEDIC DAILY ROUTINE:

The Sun is the best time to wake up Start your day early and best at the time of "Brahma muhurta" (approximately 1.5 hours prior to sunrise). The time during which sunrise occurs is thought to provide a boost of fresh vitality and energy.

Freshen and Cleanse: Begin cleansing your tongue with an instrument to scrape your tongue clean of any toxins from your mouth that are accumulated overnight. After that, you should brush your teeth, and then applying cold water to your face. Focus on your eyes. The stimulation of the senses increases circulation.

Relax: Give just a few minutes of practice of deep breathing or meditation. The time doesn't need to take long. Even 5 minutes of silence can create an ambiance of peace for your day.

Exercise Your Body: Participate with a gentle exercises. This could include a vigorous stroll, yoga or stretching. It's the idea to get blood flowing, and then get rid of any stiffness.

Eat with intention: Enjoy healthy, nutritious breakfast that's in alignment with your dosha. Pay attention to your body's signals for hunger and enjoy your food mindfully, taking in every bite.

Relax: After the day comes to an end, take time for you to unwind. Perhaps it's by relaxing with a book, listening to soothing music, or doing a easy yin yoga. Consider also self-massage using hot sesame oil. It will not only nourish the skin, but also helps prepare your body for a restful night's sleeping.

PRACTICAL EXAMPLE:

Imagine Sarah who is a 28 year old Kapha kind of. She tends to experience a lack of energy in early mornings. If she adopts an Ayurvedic regimen to start her day, she begins with a fast jog and then sipping a hot drink of tea with ginger. An invigorating beginning will keep her active and well-rested throughout the entire day.

Everyday routines are an expression of self-esteem. It's a pledge that you are important, and your health is important. As per Ayurveda the practice is a stunning practice of aligning to the natural rhythms of nature and accepting each moment with appreciation and focus.

YOGA AND MEDITATION FOR EVERY WOMAN

The modern world has embraced yoga in the form of fitness, its roots in Ayurveda and the ancient Indian theology go deeper. The essence of yoga is the fusion of body, mind, as well as the spirit. Yoga as well as meditation can be a refuge for reconnection to reenergize, re-discover yourself.

THE DUAL POWER OF YOGA AND MEDITATION:

Flexibility and physical strength The benefits of yoga include improving our physical fitness through strengthening our muscles, improving flexibility and improving posture. Particularly for women postures and asanas can provide relief from cramps during menstrual cycles, improve fertility and assist when pregnant.

Clarity of Mind and Emotional release: Meditation, when combined with yoga, can be powerful in helping to relax your mind. It helps reduce stress, anxiety and fatigue. Through focusing on breath or the specific mantra, we are able to anchor our attention to the present moment by letting go of our old regrets as well as future worries.

PERSONALIZING YOUR PRACTICE:

1. Becoming aware of your needs Understanding Your Needs: Not every yoga posture can be suitable for everyone. Pay attention to your body. If you're having menstrual issues, certain poses may not be comfortable for you. If you're pregnant, some poses might need modification. Make sure you are comfortable and security.

2. Start Small: for beginners who are new to yoga, it can be difficult to begin a 60-minute practice of yoga. Begin by taking just 10 minutes every daily. In terms of meditation, as little as 3 minutes of focused breathing could make a huge impact.

3. Find Guidance: If it's possible take a class or even workshops. The guidance of a instructor through the postures will help ensure they're done correctly and minimizes the possibility of getting injured.

PRACTICAL EXAMPLE:

Meet Maria. Maria is a mother-of-two who is in her late 30s, having a full-time job while caring for two children. In the midst of her hectic schedule, she's feeling disconnected with her own body. By introducing the practice of just 15 minutes of yoga each morning, with a focus on poses that open the heart, such as the camel (Ustrasana) or the bridge (Setu Bandhasana) and she begins your day more calm and relaxed. The addition of a five-minute meditation before the end of her day helps her rest better and helps her deal with her day's stressors.

Incorporating Ayurveda:

Yoga and Ayurveda go hand in hand. By understanding your dosha:

Vata kinds may be able to benefit from slow, grounded postures such as the Child's Pose (Balasana) or the tree pose (Vrikshasana) and when accompanied by breaths deep into the belly to ease anxiety.

A Pitta-type could concentrate on cool postures such as that of the moon salutation (Chandra Namaskar) as well as practice guided meditations using visuals to soothe their fiery nature.

Types with Kapha may require an energizing routine, such as Sun salutation (Surya Namaskar) as well as breath exercises that are energizing such as the pranayama kapalbhati.

Every woman should try yoga and meditation can be a way for one to return to the self. The goal is not to perfect a posture, but rather accepting the process, and celebrating every breath, each moment in silence, every stretch and difficulty. It's a lifetime practice of self-awareness, self-love and awareness.

Mindful Living: From Consumption to Relationships In the rapid-paced society It's easy to get distracted and not take the time to stop for reflection, ponder, and take in the present. Mindful living refers to the deliberate practice of being fully present all the time in our life. Through mindfulness you not only improve your experiences of life, as well as improve the quality of our emotional and mental well-being. This practice is in full alignment with the holistic approach to the world.

MINDFULNESS IN CONSUMPTION:

Start by observing what you are eating. Do you find it nutritious or empty? Do you eat quickly or taking moment to take the time to appreciate each bite? Instead eating a mindless snack during a show you should sit down to appreciate its texture, flavor, as well as how your feel. Select foods that are healthy and balanced with your dosha.

Consumption: In the midst of endless advertisement and consumption, you should consider before making a purchase: "Do I truly need this?" Opt to buy quality products over mass. Choose sustainable brands and environmentally friendly choices that align with the Ayurvedic philosophy of harmony with the natural world.

MINDFULNESS IN DAILY ACTIVITIES:

Active listening: No matter if you are having a conversation with your partner or playing music be sure to be active in your listening. That means staying fully engaged and taking in the meaning and not letting your thoughts wander.

Routine tasks Simple tasks such as dishwashing or cleaning could be transformed into a state of meditational. Take a bath, feel the water, watch the bubbles of soap, observe how you breathing. When completely embraced, are an uplifting and calming experience.

MINDFUL RELATIONSHIPS:

Present: The greatest present you can offer anyone is the complete attention of your. While with family and friends make sure you are attentive. Disconnect from distractions like smartphones and have deep conversation.

"Empathy and Understanding" When you are in a disagreement rather than reacting quickly and impulsively, breathe deeply and seek to be able to see your opponent's point of view. React with compassion and kindness.

Self-reflection: Spend the time to get to know your self. Find out the triggers you are experiencing and what patterns you have within your relationships. Are you bringing past baggage into current interactions? Introspection and mindfulness can heal the wounds of the past and build better interactions.

Practical Example:

Meet Aisha. After several failed relationships, she chose to go on a retreat for mindfulness. She learned how to be aware and noticed that she was often carrying the burden of previous betrayals into relationships that made these relationships strained right from the beginning. Through every day meditation and journaling, Aisha started healing the old marks. Aisha now approach relationships by opening her mind and body, which eventually leads to stronger relationships.

HOLISTIC MINDFULNESS:

Ayurveda shows us that all things are interconnected. Our bodies, minds and our souls are all connected to everything that surrounds us. When we are mindful, we do not only enhance our personal experience but we also help create an environment that is more peaceful. This is an effect that ripples. When we consume with conscious thought and sustainably, we are promoting sustainable living. When we are in a relationship by expressing love and compassion that promote peace and harmony.

NATURAL DETOX AND REJUVENATION TECHNIQUES

Our daily routines mean that we're confronted with a myriad of external contaminants, ranging including polluted air and processed food items. In the internal, stress and negative emotions may build up as emotional and mental toxic substances. Ayurveda has a wide range of methods for rejuvenation and detoxification which not only purify the body, but also renew the soul and mind.

DIGESTIVE FIRE (AGNI) AND ITS ROLE IN DETOX:

In the midst of Ayurvedic detox is the idea of Agni or which is the digestion fire. A healthy Agni is able to efficiently process foods, making sure that nutrients are taken in and that toxins (known in the form of Ama) are eliminated. But a weakened Agni causes the build-up of Ama which can cause a variety of ailments. Constantly stimulating and maintaining your Agni is crucial to efficient detoxification.

Toxifying your body by Diet:

Fasting Ayurveda recommends occasional fasting, or light eating in order to allow the digestive system to take an opportunity to rest and allow for an organic cleansing. It doesn't mean completely abstinence from eating, but rather opting to eat lighter, easy to digest meals such as Khichdi (a combination of lentils and rice) as well as warm vegetable broths.

Included Detoxifying Foods in your Diet foods like ginger as well as turmeric and fenugreek have the ability to naturally enhance the process of detoxification in your body. Incorporating these into your diet could help support an easy and continuous cleansing.

REJUVENATION WITH AYURVEDIC PRACTICES:

Abhyanga (Ayurvedic oil Massage) Full-body massage that is performed using warming, medicinal oils will not only help relax your body, but assists in removing toxic substances. Abhyanga massages regularly can help improve complexion texture, increase circulation and increase general vitality.

Swedana (Herbal Steam Therapy) after the oil massage, steam therapy may aid in opening the pores and helping to eliminate toxins that have accumulated via sweat.

Neti as well as Nasya Nasya: They are both methods for cleansing the nasal passages. When Neti is the process of cleaning the nasal passages by using saline waters, Nasya is the administration of herbs or oils that are medicated via the nose. These methods can aid in removing nasal congestion, improving breathing health and the mental clarity.

MENTAL AND EMOTIONAL REJUVENATION:

Meditation: A daily practice of practice of meditation does not just calm the mind but can also assist in the release of emotional burdens. Strategies like mindfulness meditation and the chanting of mantras can be especially efficient.

Pranayama (Breathing exercises) Pranayama: Exercises such as Anulom-Vilom (alternate nostril breath) as well as Kapalbhati (rapid breath exhalation) will help to oxygenate your body, boost mental focus as well as create a feeling of peace within.

Practical Example:

Meet Rohan. He would feel tired at midday and suffer from constant headaches, which impeded his performance. Conscient of the need for detoxification the following week, he started a diet of fasting, eating just teas and fruits on a Saturday. The morning routine was also initiated by taking a 10 minute Anulom-Vilom and a brief time of meditation. In the course of a few several weeks, his levels of energy increased, and headaches were no longer a problem. The detoxification process did more than just rejuvenate his body, but also brought greater clarity in his thinking.

Implementing techniques for rejuvenation and detoxification does not require a major life-style change. Simple, routine actions, if practiced consistently are able to bring about dramatic transformations, reviving and uplifting yourself from within.

Chapter 9: Emotional And Spiritual Flourishing

THE MIND-BODY CONNECTION IN AYURVEDA

The wisdom from the ancient times of Ayurveda acknowledges the vital connection with the mind as well as body. In contrast to the simplistic view of wellness in many modern-day methods, Ayurveda views the individual as an entire person, covering both the physical and emotional. Each cell of the body responds to thinking, while your brain is able to sense the echo of the experiences your body has.

Sattva, Rajas, and Tamas in Ayurveda the three gunas (qualities) represent our mental state. Sattva symbolizes pureness and wisdom, Rajas represents action and motion, and Tamas represents inertia as well as darkness. Sattvic states are perfect for spiritual development and mental focus.

The Seven Chakras: Ayurveda acknowledges seven energy centers within our bodies, which align with the spine. They are referred to as chakras. Each chakra corresponds with certain bodily functions as well as emotions. A healthy balance between these chakras will affect physical health as well as the emotional state of being.

PRACTICES TO OVERCOME STRESS AND ANXIETY

Anxiety and stress can be manifested as physical discomfort and emotional tension. Ayurveda offers a variety of methods to help restore equilibrium:

Abhyanga (Self-Massage) massaging your body using warm oil such as coconut, sesame, or can be a practice of grounding which can ease anxiety. It is especially beneficial when performed prior to bedtime in order to encourage peaceful sleep.

Pranayama (Breath Control) techniques such as anulom and vilom (alternate nostril breathing) are a great way to relax your mind, enhancing the concentration of your mind, as well as reducing anxiety.

Ayurvedic Herbs Ashwagandha as well as Brahmi are two plants that are often suggested to fight stress. They aid in reviving the body and boost resilience to anxiety.

DEEPENING SELF-AWARENESS AND SPIRITUAL GROWTH

Ayurveda believes in the fundamental capacity of self-understanding. When we connect with our own inner self it is possible to achieve peace within our world.

Meditation: Everyday mindfulness, even if it's for only a few minutes, is able to be a significant improvement. Meditation can help in increasing awareness of oneself, increasing concentration as well as connecting to one's spiritual self.

Dinacharya (Daily routine) An ongoing schedule that is in line with the rhythms of nature will keep both the mind and body in top state. It includes getting up early, eating regularly and a bed time that is early.

Study of sacred texts The study of scriptures or other spiritual texts can give us profound insight and help us to stay grounded when we are in a state of chaos.

TOOLS FOR RESILIENCE AND JOY

The qualities of resilience and happiness don't have to be just things that happen to people They can be nurtured. Ayurveda offers a variety of tools to bring joy into your life:

Gratitude Journal: Daily noting your gratitude for things could help shift your focus away off of what's missing or negative about your life and instead focus on the abundance you already have in your life.

Connecting to Nature Being outdoors, be it the forests, riversides or mountains can rejuvenate your mind and soul.

Nurturing Relationships and keeping Sattvic (harmonious) relations with people close to you is not only a source of emotional support but also increases your the mental and spiritual resiliency.

Dance and Music Involving with activities that lift spirits, like dancing or listening to music that lifts the spirit, dancing can bring happiness and diminish emotions of sadness, or heavyness.

Be aware that while Ayurveda provides a variety of methods, it's important to discover what resonates with your personal preferences.

Chapter 10: Navigating The World Of Ayurvedic Herbs

MOST COMMONLY USED HERBS FOR WOMEN'S HEALTH

Ayurveda has a wide range of medicinal herbs to address different aspects of women's health. The most important herbs comprise:

Shatavari (Asparagus racemosus) is often referred to as"the "Queen of Herbs," Shatavari aids in promoting fertility, improves reproductive health and acts as a rejuvenating supplement for female health.

Ashwagandha (Withania somnifera) known for its adaptogenic qualities that help to combat anxiety, increases vitality and aids in maintaining the balance of hormones.

Amla (Emblica officinalis) A powerful food source of Vitamin C helps to improve healthy skin and hair. It also boosts immunity and helps digestion.

Turmeric (Curcuma longa) is known for its anti-inflammatory properties, it's an absolute beneficial for skin and helps menstrual health by alleviating menstrual cramps.

Triphala is a combination of three fruit - Amla, Haritaki, and Bibhitaki It's a soft detoxifier that promotes digestion health and health.

DOS AND DON'TS OF HERBAL CONSUMPTION

Although Ayurvedic herbs may be powerful and effective, they should be used with care:

"Consultation: Always seek the advice of an knowledgeable Ayurvedic practitioner prior to beginning any regimen of herbs.

Be sure to follow the recommended dosages It's not always the case that more is better. Be sure to adhere to the dosages prescribed for avoiding potential negative side consequences.

Beware of self-diagnosis. It's tempting to prescribe herbs by self-based from research on the internet, but it's never safe.

Listen to your body If any herbal remedy makes you feel sick or experience adverse reactions, discontinue your consumption and speak with an expert.

INTERACTIONS WITH MODERN PHARMACEUTICALS

Similar to modern medications, Ayurvedic herbs can have interaction with

Be Educated When you're using an medications that are allopathic, tell your Ayurvedic physician about the medication in order to prevent possible interactions.

Staggering Consumption: As an overall guideline If you're consuming both Ayurvedic herbalism and modern medical treatments attempt to space out your consumption for a couple of hours.

Awareness and Research Certain herbs may enhance or block the effects of drugs. Keep yourself informed and stay vigilant.

PURCHASING AND STORING HERBS

The effectiveness of Ayurvedic herbs is largely dependent on the quality of their ingredients:

"Certified Suppliers": Buy herbal products only from reliable and certified suppliers in order to assure the authenticity and pureness of your herbs.

Make sure to check expiry dates. Although Ayurvedic herbs may seem organic as they are evergreen and a natural source of nutrition, they do have shelves that last for a while. Always check expiration dates.

Storage: Keep the herbs in a cool and dry area, preferring airtight containers. Be sure to protect them from sun, water, and bugs.

Do not use plastic: If you can, do not store herb in plastic containers. Glass and stainless steel containers are preferred since they protect the purity and potency of the herb.

Keep in mind that, even though Ayurveda provides the bounty of nature through the use of plants, eating them in a responsible manner will ensure their health benefits and protects from potential hazards.

Chapter 11: Ayurvedic Nutrition

Food is regarded as medicine in Ayurveda as well as a healthy diet is crucial to ensure good health. The chapter in this section will look at the fundamentals of Ayurvedic diet, which stress the importance of eating mindfully along with seasonal and seasonal meals, as well as eating a balanced and healthy food plan.

The seven tastes and their effects on doshas. We also provide the necessary guidelines to create nourishing and nourishing food items. By utilizing Ayurvedic food, we can develop a positive connection with food, and tap into its therapeutic potential.

Ayurvedic Lifestyle Tips Ayurveda gives a broad guideline for living a healthy and fulfilled life. This chapter will dive into the many lifestyle choices that are recommended by Ayurveda to promote overall wellbeing. From our daily routines (Dinacharya) to the seasonal rituals (Ritucharya) We explore the ways that aligning our choices in life to the natural rhythms improves our health and enhance longevity. The discussion also focuses on the importance of exercise, sleep as well as stress management to maintain the health and vitality of our lives.

Ayurvedic Detoxification

The body's toxins build up as time passes, causing problems for the efficient performance of our biological system. Ayurveda acknowledges the necessity of a regular cleanse to remove the impurities and restore equilibrium. In this article we will explore the fundamentals and methods in Ayurvedic detoxification. The chapter focuses on Panchakarma known as the most renowned Ayurvedic detoxification therapy along with different detoxification techniques which can easily be incorporated in our lives. When we embrace Ayurvedic detoxification, it is possible to refresh our mind, body and soul.

Ayurvedic herbal Remedies Herbs play a crucial part in Ayurvedic medical practices, providing safe and efficient solutions to various problems with health. In this article we will explore the vast world of Ayurvedic herbs as well as their therapeutic qualities. We explore the Ayurvedic pharmacycopeia, focusing on the most commonly-used herbs and their uses.

Additionally, we offer guidance regarding how to make herbal remedies safe and efficiently. Utilizing the strength of Ayurvedic herbalism, we will be able to aid in our overall health and bring back the balance.

Ayurvedic home remedies for skin and Hair. Radiant, healthy glowing skin and beautiful hair reflect the your inner health and vitality. Ayurveda provides a wealth of practices and remedies that nourish and revive the beauty of our exterior. In this section we look at Ayurvedic solutions for home use to treat skincare and hair treatment. The range of products includes natural face masks, herbs for hair oils to revitalizing self-massage, we will discover how to glow complexion and shiny hair. Through embracing Ayurvedic practices for beauty and practices, we will improve the appearance of our body while promoting the holistic health.

Ayurvedic remedies for common ailments Ayurveda offers a wide array of cures for the most common ailments and enables people to manage their health on their own. In this section we will explore Ayurvedic solutions for common issues with your health. From colds and digestive issues to sleep disorders and headaches The chapter discusses practical remedies drawn of Ayurvedic wisdom. Utilizing these tried-and-true treatments, we are able to treat small ailments, and encourage self-healing.

Ayurvedic remedies for women's health Ayurveda is aware of the specific female health issues and provides specialized treatments for many female-related ailments. In this chapter, we dive into Ayurvedic treatments to improve women's health. This includes hormone imbalances, menstrual problems as well as menopausal symptoms.

We explore the idea that menstrual health is an indicator of overall health and examine natural ways of helping women through different phases of their life. In accepting Ayurvedic treatments for women's wellbeing and balance, women are able to achieve harmony as well as vitality and empower.

Ayurvedic Yoga practices for Harmony and harmony Ayurveda and yoga can be described as twin science that can complement one another in a seamless way. This chapter will dive into the interplay between Ayurveda and yoga, examining the synergistic advantages of these ancient techniques. There are particular yoga poses (poses) and pranayama (breathing exercises) as well as meditation methods which are in line with Ayurvedic concepts. Through integrating Ayurvedic yoga techniques into our schedule, we will be able to cultivate stability, flexibility, and harmony within ourselves.

Ayurvedic Approach to Mental Well-being Ayurveda acknowledges the significance of maintaining mental health to maintain the overall wellbeing and health. The chapter we are discussing will look at the Ayurvedic method of fostering an unwinding and well-balanced mind. The chapter explores Ayurvedic herbal remedies, diet recommendations and practices for living which promote clarity of mind mental stability, emotional balance, and reduce stress. When we adopt Ayurvedic techniques for mental wellbeing to achieve peace and a resilient mental state.

Ayurvedic treatments and therapeutic modalities Ayurveda is a vast array of treatments and healing techniques which go far beyond the traditional herbal cure. In this chapter we look at Ayurvedic treatments like Abhyanga (Ayurvedic massage), Shirodhara (oil pouring onto foreheads) as well as Pinda Sweda (herbal massage using bolus). Additionally, we will look at Ayurvedic methods for rejuvenation such as Rasayana and Marma treatment. When embracing these treatments, people can enjoy profound relaxation, revitalization, and re-energization of vital energy.

Ayurveda for Children and Family Health 5

Ayurveda offers valuable information as well as guidelines to improve well-being and health of kids and families. In this section we will discuss Ayurvedic strategies for pediatric health which include diet recommendations along with herbal remedies and lifestyle habits that are tailored specifically to the demands of children. Also, we examine Ayurvedic concepts that help support families' health and wellbeing, which includes mindful food choices, healthy relationships, as well as healthy routines for daily life. Through integrating Ayurvedic knowledge into our family lives it is possible to promote healthy and well-being for each member of the family.

Ayurveda to prolong life and aging smoothly Ayurveda gives profound insights about the aging process and how to cultivate longevity. In the final chapter it explores Ayurvedic methods that promote an age-related healthy lifestyle and smooth passage through the various phases of life. The chapter discusses Rasayana (rejuvenation) treatments along with dietary suggestions and lifestyle habits that help to increase the vitality of our brains and general well-being in the midst of aging. Through embracing Ayurvedic practices for longevity and health, people will live their lives with vitality, grace as well as a sensation of happiness.

Ayurveda, the oldest holistic system of healing that originated of the Indian subcontinent is an incredible treasure trove of knowledge that has stood the tests of the passage of. Its history spans over five thousand years

For thousands of years, Ayurveda provides an extensive way to improve health and well-being and wellness, not only focusing on the physical, but the mental, emotional as well as spiritual aspects of human life.

The word "Veda" comes from Sanskrit word "Ayur" (life) and "Veda"

(knowledge or (knowledge or), Ayurveda is often called the

"Science of Life." It's based on the basic premise that human bodies are an integral part of the larger universe. It is linked to the rhythms and natural elements. In understanding and aligning the natural forces that surround us, Ayurveda empowers individuals to maintain balance, avoid disease and improve longevity.

The central concept of Ayurveda is the idea of three doshas, Vata, Pitta, and Kapha. These three doshas are the core biochemical forces, or energy sources that control the physical and mental processes in the human body. Every person is believed to be an individual combination of these doshas that is what determines their unique constitution, also known as Prakriti. Through understanding the individual's Prakriti Ayurveda offers personalised advice on diet, lifestyle and treatments for therapeutic purposes for maintaining the best health possible.

The holistic aspect of Ayurveda transcends the body's physical structure.

It acknowledges the complex connection between mind, body and spirit. It emphasizes the significance of mental and emotional health in general wellbeing. Ayurveda believes that the mind is an extremely powerful 8

The force that determines our condition of health, and play crucially in the control and prevention of illnesses. Methods like meditation, yoga, as well as mindfulness are incorporated into Ayurvedic techniques to help promote psychological clarity and harmony and spiritual growth.

It also focuses heavily on the importance of preventive health. It acknowledges that the primary reason for illness is often in the buildup of imbalances and toxins in the mind and body.

With various detoxification techniques including diet and other lifestyle changes, Ayurveda aims to remove these imbalances and restore your body's natural healing capabilities. Through an approach that is proactive to their health, people will be able to lower the likelihood of developing illness, and also maintain their health.

The therapies offered of Ayurveda can be vast and wide-ranging that range from herbal treatments and diet adjustments, to more specialized treatment and rejuvenation treatments. Ayurvedic practitioners draw on an extensive list of medicinal herbs and minerals carefully selected and used to correct particular imbalances or conditions. They believe that these natural cures to function in harmony with the body and promote the healing process and helping restore balance, with no harmful adverse negative side effects.

In addition, Ayurveda recognizes the unique demands on health for every stage of life. It offers recommendations for postnatal and prenatal health, the development of children as well as the difficulties and transitions that occur during the various stages of adulthood as well as old years. In honoring the natural cycles and alterations of life Ayurveda provides insights and techniques to ensure optimal wellbeing throughout the entire life cycle.

Recent years have seen Ayurveda has been recognized and gained recognition across the Western world for its alternative, complementary and holistic alternative to conventional medicine. The holistic principles of Ayurveda and its traditional therapies are a perfect match for 9

and those looking for a customized and integrated method of health and wellness. But it's important to remember that Ayurveda does not substitute of modern medicine. It is instead considered a complement to conventional medicine that is used in conjunction with traditional medicine in order to offer an integrated and holistic treatment for wellness.

The Mind-Body Connection of Ayurveda Ayurveda The ancient science of living, acknowledges the unbreakable link between body and mind. The chapter in this article will will explore the deep understanding of relationship between the mind and body in Ayurveda and the implications it has to our well-being and health.

Ayurveda considers the body and mind as two distinct aspects of us, continuously impacting and shaping one another. The condition of our minds influences the overall health of our bodies, in the same way because the overall health of our bodies affects the calmness and strength of our thoughts. The holistic approach is aware that true wellness cannot be realized until both your body and mind are in equilibrium.

According to Ayurveda is comprised of three primary qualities also known as Gunas: Sattva, Rajas Tamas, and Tamas. Sattva symbolizes purity, clearness and harmony. It's associated with attributes like peace, happiness and sagacity. Rajas symbolize energy, activity as well as passion. It's associated with characteristics like restlessness, ambition and craving. Tamas is a symbol of inertia, dark and weight. It's associated with traits such as apathy, lethargy and illusion.

When your mind is in the state of Sattva the mind is at peace clear and open to wisdom and higher levels of knowledge. The state of mind promotes positive feelings as well as mental clarity and an overall sense of wellbeing. However the moment your mind is overruled through Rajas or Tamas and Tamas, the mind can become unstable, confused and more prone to negativity and disturbances.

Ayurveda believes that the mind is affected by many aspects, such as our emotions, thoughts as well as sensory experiences and our overall physical and mental health. It stresses the importance of fostering an optimistic mental state and fostering positive emotions as well as engaging in activities which promote clarity of mind and balance in our emotions.

One of the most important techniques that is used in Ayurveda to strengthen the body-mind connection is meditation. Meditation can help us relax your mind, develop self-awareness, and tap into our own wisdom.

By regularly practicing meditation We can lower anxiety, improve the mental health of our clients, and increase an overall sense of inner calm and peace.

Ayurveda is also aware of the effects of lifestyle and diet on our minds. What we eat has directly influenced our mood. Ayurvedic food recommendations emphasize eating healthy, fresh foods which are nutritious and digestible. An energizing diet that contains abundant fresh vegetables, fruits and other fruit as well as whole grains and healthy fats is beneficial for functioning of the brain and well-being.

Apart from eating habits, Ayurveda emphasizes the importance for a well-balanced everyday routine. It is also called Dinacharya. Maintaining a regular daily schedule assists in synchronizing our bodily rhythms and fosters a sense of harmony and stability. It involves practices like getting up early, doing gentle exercises as well as meditation and meals. When we align our day-to-day routines with the rhythms of our day, we can establish the perfect environment to have that healthy body and mind.

Ayurveda acknowledges the effect of external elements in our mental health. Sensory experiences including what we feel, see or hear, feel or taste are able to significantly affect the state of our mind 12

of the mind. Ayurveda is a way to fill us with positive and harmonious spaces, and engage in actions which bring joy to our lives and avoid the exposure to harmful influence.

In addition, Ayurveda acknowledges the role of our emotions on our general well-being. Insufferable emotional patterns and stress may cause imbalances within the body and mind. Ayurveda offers a variety of methods for relaxation and emotional cleansing such as breathing exercises as well as herbal therapies Aromatherapy, as well as therapies that are therapeutic, such as Shirodhara (oil applying over forehead) as well as Abhyanga (Ayurvedic oil massage).

Knowing the Doshas In Ayurveda, the doshas are the energy sources which control our physical as well as psychological functions. Knowing the doshas is essential to understanding our individual body and the ways how imbalances may influence the health of our body. This chapter will look at the three doshas - Vata, Pitta and Kapha. We also look at their functions, characteristics as well as their impact on our health and well-being.

Vata Dosha:

Vata is the dosha which has been associated to the components of space and air. Vata is a symbol of change, movement as well as creativity.

People who have dominant Vata nature tend to possess a slim physique, speedy and smooth moves, as well as a lively temperament. They're often creative energetic, awe-inspiring, and subject to a variety of mental and physical dimensions.

If Vata is at its best it encourages vitality physical agility, mental acuity, and flexibility. But, an over- or imbalance in Vata may cause a myriad of problems with health, like insomnia, anxiety, digestion issues, joint pains and other. In order to balance Vata it is recommended to adhere to a schedule and engage in activities that calm such as meditation or gentle exercise and eat warming, nutritious food items.

Pitta Dosha:

Pitta is connected to elemental elements like fire as well as water. Pitta embodies qualities like the transformation of metabolism, change and the intensity.

People who have a dominant Pitta constitution typically possess an average of 14

moderate build, an incisive brain, and an intense desire to achieve.

They can be driven, focused and are able to lead.

If Pitta is balanced It promotes digestive health, mental clarity and the ability to focus. An excess or unbalanced Pitta could manifest as irritation, anger as well as digestive problems.

In order to balance Pitta people should practice moderate consumption to engage in activities that cool and eat foods that cool you down, and control stress efficiently.

Kapha Dosha:

Kapha is related to the earth element and water. It represents the virtues of durability, stability and caring.

People who have a dominant Kapha constitution usually are strong, have with a serene disposition and an empathetic temperament. They're generally solid, supportive and intolerant of changes.

If Kapha is balanced it enhances resilience, stability, and well-being. In contrast, an over- or imbalance in Kapha could cause lethargy as well as weight gain, congestion as well as a sense of an emotional attachment. To maintain balance Kapha people are encouraged to regularly exercise as well as follow a schedule that is stimulating eating light and warm meals, and build the sense of purpose and a sense of enthusiasm.

It is crucial to remember that every person has an individual combination of these doshas. They are referred to by the Prakriti which is also known as their constitution. Being aware of the individual's Prakriti can provide personalized suggestions as well as interventions that help to keep or bring balance back. A qualified Ayurvedic practitioner is able to identify the individual's Prakriti by conducting a thorough examination of both psychological and physical characteristics, lifestyle variables as well as health histories.

Apart from Prakriti The Ayurvedic system also acknowledges the impact of external influences upon the doshas. The factors that are known as Vikruti and Vikruti, are the state that is currently in imbalance or doshic balance. Through analyzing each of Prakriti along with Vikruti, Ayurvedic practitioners can create customized treatments, nutritional guidelines, as well as lifestyle modifications to correct imbalances and bring back harmony.

Chapter 12: Understanding Agni Digestive Fire

Agni also known as the digestive fire, lies central to Ayurvedic nutrition. It is the body's capacity to absorb and digest foods. If Agni is in good health it is able to ensure effective digestion, absorption and elimination. But, if Agni is in poor health or imbalanced is imbalanced, it could lead to problems with digestion, nutrient deficiencies, as well as the build-up of the toxins (ama) within the body.

Ayurveda stresses the importance of burning and maintaining a healthy Agni through diet as well as mindful eating. That means eating food items that are easy to digest as well as eating according to regular meals eating a balanced diet, and not overeating and eating even when you're not hungry.

The Six Tastes:

Ayurveda acknowledges the six flavors that can be found in different dishes such as sweet, sour, bitter, salty and an astringent. Each flavor has distinct characteristics and affects the doshas in a different way. In a balanced diet, it is recommended to contain all six of the tastes in the right proportions so as to keep doshic equilibrium.

Sweet flavor (Madhura) Sweet taste (Madhura): The sweetness of the taste encourages groundedness, nourishment and satisfaction. It is present in many foods like cereal grains, sweet fruit dairy products, as well as natural sweeteners such as honey. But, the excessive consumption of sweet foods may increase Kapha dosha levels and cause an increase in weight and fatigue.

Taste of sour (Amla) Sour taste (Amla): It stimulates digestion and gives a sweet taste. It can be located in the citrus fruits, as well as food products that are fermented, as well as vinegar. A moderate intake of sour food are a good way to help balance Vata dosha. However, over consumption could cause Pitta dosha and cause inflammation and acidity.

Salty flavor (Lavana) Salty taste improves the flavor and helps to maintain healthy water balance within the body. It can be found in sea and salty vegetables and certain dairy items. In excess, however, salt consumption could cause the retention of fluids and cause imbalances in Pitta as well as Kapha doshas.

Bitter flavor (Tikta) Bitter taste helps in cleansing, detoxification as well as cooling. It can be found in green leafy vegetables, herbal extracts like neem and turmeric as well as bitter melons. The bitter taste of foods may help to balance Pitta as well as Kapha doshas. However, over consumption can boost Vata dosha, which can cause dryness.

The taste of pungency (Katu) Its strong taste of the spice stimulates digestion, circulation and warm. It is present in many spice like chili peppers, black pepper and ginger. Intoxicating foods can help balance Kapha as well as Vata doshas however they must be eaten in moderation because they may aggravate Pitta dosha, which can cause inflammation.

Astringent tastes (Kashaya) The astringent taste is drying and has a the effect of tightening. It is present in many foods such as legumes, green tea as well as certain fruit like the pomegranate.

Astringent foods may help to balance Pitta as well as Kapha doshas. However, the excessive consumption of these foods can raise Vata dosha and lead to dryness.

Individualized Dietary Recommendations for Health: Ayurveda acknowledges that every person has their own unique constitution, and thus requires different dietary suggestions. The three doshas Vata, Pitta, and Kapha each have their own diets and dietary guidelines that help ensure harmony.

Vata Pacifying Diet: For those who have the dominant Vata constitution or who are experiencing Vata imbalances the Vata-pacifying food plan is suggested. It includes cooked, warm meals, oil-rich foods as well as grounding spices and sweet, sour and salty flavours. Affirming against cold or raw food as well as excessive caffeine and lighter, dry foods are equally beneficial.

Pitta-Pacifying Diet: People who have an overt Pitta health or Pitta imbalances need to adopt a Pitta-pacifying regimen. This means eating cooling and hydrating food items, abstaining from extreme heat or spicy food as well as focusing on sweetness, bitterness, and astringent flavours. Fresh vegetables, fruits as well as whole grains and herbaceous plants like coriander and fennel can be helpful.

A diet that is Kapha-pacifying for people who have a predominant Kapha body or Kapha imbalances the Kapha-pacifying diet is suggested. It includes light and warming dishes, foods that contain strong and bitter taste in addition to avoiding excessively oily and sweet food items. Consuming a wide variety of veggies or legumes as well as grain-based foods is suggested.

Mindful Eating Practices:

Ayurveda insists on the importance of eating mindfully to aid digestion and maintain doshic equilibrium. A few of the most significant practices are:

Dining in a tranquil and tranquil environment, away from the distractions.

Foods should be chewed thoroughly in order to improve digestion and absorption of nutrients.

Stay clear of eating too much and listen to your body's signals of fullness and hunger.

eating meals regularly to create a regular routine and to help Agni.

The Role of Food Combinations:

It also stresses the importance of various food groups to help support proper digestion and stop the creation of toxic substances (ama). The right food combination can increase digestion and help prevent discomfort. Some general guidelines include:

Avoiding food mixtures that may be incompatible like mixing sour fruit and milk or mixing fish and milk.

Fruits should be eaten separately from other food items, preferring to eat them with a full stomach, or in snacks.

Blending different foods that have similar digestive characteristics to help ensure effective digestion.

In adhering to these fundamentals of Ayurvedic diet and making mindful choices about how we eat will help to maintain the doshic balance, improve digestion and wellbeing overall. In the next section we'll explore Ayurvedic habits that can complement our diets and aid in maintaining our health and vitality.

Ayurvedic Lifestyle practices Ayurveda isn't just regarding diet choices, it is an entire health and wellness system that covers a variety of aspects of our lives. In this article we explore Ayurvedic life practices that go along with our dietary habits and help us maintain our health and vitality. They include routines for daily life as well as self-care routines as well as mindful practices to help aid in harmony, balance and general well-being.

Daily Routine (Dinacharya):Ayurveda emphasizes the importance of following a daily routine to synchronize our activities with the natural rhythms of the day. A structured daily routine helps to maintain the equilibrium of the doshas, and improves our mental and physical capabilities. The most important components of a regular routine are:

Early rise: waking up earlier than sunrise lets us be in tune with the tranquil and revitalizing aspects of the early morning.

Scraping your tongue: Gently scraping your tongue using the tongue scraper after waking assists in removing toxins and improves digestion.

Dental hygiene: Cleaning the gums and teeth, in conjunction with oil pulling, help keep oral health in check and encourages cleansing.

Self-massage (Abhyanga) Massage the body using warm oil prior to showering can help relax and hydrate the skin and strengthens the lymphatic organs.

Showering or bath can help cleanse your body and revive your senses.

Breathing and meditation exercises Meditation and deep breathing or pranayama exercises during the early morning hours improves concentration, relieves anxiety, and helps to cultivate the feeling of peace within.

Regular exercise: Engaging in physical exercise, for example walking, yoga or any other form of exercise that improves endurance, circulation and the flexibility.

Food intake at regular times: Having regularly at the same time supports digestion and helps maintain a healthy metabolism.

Time to go to bed earlier will allow adequate rest and rejuvenation throughout the evening.

Mindfulness and Stress Management:

Ayurveda recognizes the effect of stress on overall wellbeing.

The stress of being stressed out can alter the balance of doshic hormones and lead to health concerns of various kinds. So, including meditation and techniques for stress reduction to our everyday lives is essential. A few of these practices include:

Mindfulness awareness: Maintaining a state of present awareness allows us to stay in touch with our body, the mind and our emotions helping to improve self-reflection as well as the reduction of stress.

Techniques for relaxation and meditation Meditation either guided imagery, meditation, or progressive techniques to relax muscles will help calm your mind, ease anxiety and help to maintain emotional equilibrium.

Gentle exercise and yoga Involving in yoga poses as well as gentle stretching and other

161

types of exercise, does not only improve physically but can also improve psychological and mental well-being.

Connecting with nature The act of spending time outdoors in the natural world such as strolls in the park garden, or being in a chair for 22 hours.

Outdoors, it helps to restore equilibrium, ease stress and encourages a sense balance with the natural world.

Journaling A journal is a way to express oneself as well as reflection as well as emotional processing.

Sleep Hygiene:

A restful and adequate sleep is crucial to maintain health and balance in the doshic system as well as overall wellbeing. Ayurveda gives advice on how to establish regular and healthy sleeping practices. A few suggestions include:

Establishing a peaceful nighttime routine by engaging in calming activities like reading, relaxing in a warm bath or doing gently stretching prior to bed will help get your body and mind ready to sleep.

Refrain from engaging in stimulating activities just before sleeping: limiting the exposure to screens on electronic devices or intense conversations, as well as stimulant drinks like coffee during the night helps to ensure the peaceful transition to sleeping.

Designing a sleeping environment The creation of a cozy, dark and peaceful sleep space encourages restful and peaceful sleeping.

Regularly sleeping schedules Sleeping and getting up at the same intervals supports the body's normal cycles of circadian rhythms. It also improves sleeping quality.

Self-care Rituals:

Ayurveda stresses self-care practices to nurture and nourish us on an emotional, physical mental, and spiritual scale. Some self-care practices include:

Massage with oil (Abhyanga) Massaging regularly your body with warm oil does not just help with physical health, but it also encourages the sense of relaxation, self-love, as well as acceptance of oneself.

Skin care: Utilizing natural and healthy products for your skin that are appropriate for your skin type will help to maintain a healthy, vibrant and youthful skin.

Gentle detoxification methods: Integrating techniques like saunas, dry brushing steam baths, or herbal steam are a great way to aid in detoxification and revitalization.

Mindful eating: The practice of mindful eating, enjoying every bite, and developing gratitude for what that we get supports an enlightened relationship with food, and helps to promote optimal digestion.

Involvement in pursuits that make you smile like artistic pursuits, hobbies or spending time with your family members, or engaging in religious practices that nourish the soul, and boosts general well-being.

Incorporating the Ayurvedic practice in our everyday lives and practices, we can build an environment of harmony and support that promotes our well-being and health. In the next section we'll explore Ayurvedic detox methods that can help eliminate toxins and increase health and vitality.

Ayurvedic detoxification and cleansing is an essential element of Ayurvedic health and well-being. In this article we will explore Ayurvedic detoxification techniques that assist to detoxify the body, eliminate the accumulation of toxins (ama) as well as boost the health of your body. These methods aim to help support our body's naturally detoxification mechanisms and bring balance to the both the mental and physical emotional levels.

Understanding Ama:

According to Ayurveda Ama is a toxic substance that builds up in your body because of insufficient digestion, unhealthy life choices as well as environmental influences. Ama is believed to be a key factor in a variety of health conditions and imbalances. Ayurvedic detoxification techniques concentrate on removing ama as well as restoring the body's tissue and organs.

Panchakarma:

Panchakarma is an internationally acclaimed Ayurvedic treatment for rejuvenation and detoxification. It's a full-service treatment that includes a variety of rejuvenating and cleansing therapies that are tailored to each person's individual health and lifestyle. The typical panchakarma session consists of five main methods:

Vamana is a therapeutic emesis that helps remove excessive Kapha and other toxins out of the upper tract of the gastrointestinal.

Virechana: Therapeutic purgation that helps rid Pitta-related toxins of the gallbladder, the liver, as well as the intestines.

Basti: Herbal enemas that detox the colon and to balance Vata dosha.

Nasya is the nasal administration of powders or oils made from herbs to remove toxic substances from the head and neck area.

Rakta Mokshana: Bloodletting, or the therapeutic cleansing of blood to eliminate impure blood.

Panchakarma is done under the supervision of an experienced Ayurvedic practitioner. It provides the deepest detoxification, revitalization as well as restoring balance. It's recommended for people suffering from specific health problems or as a preventative measure for overall health.

Chapter 13: Dietary Detoxification

Ayurveda stresses the importance of food in helping detoxification.

Certain Ayurvedic food practices that help in rejuvenation and cleansing are:

Fasting: A short-term or modified fasting allows for the digestive system to rest, and aids in the elimination of the toxins. Fasting must be conducted under the supervision of a qualified professional.

Easy to digest and light-weight foods easy to digest: A diet that is primarily plant-based, organic seasonally available, and prepared with digestive spices aids in digestion and cleansing. Refraining from processed, heavy and difficult to digest foods can be beneficial for detoxification.

Herbal teas and infusions The consumption of herbal teas or infusions comprised of herbs that detoxify like turmeric, ginger as well as dandelion and cilantro aids in the body's natural detoxification functions.

Incorporating detoxifying ingredients like cumin, coriander and fennel as well as fenugreek during cooking help to improve digestion, aid in the elimination of toxins, and help to balance the doshas.

Hydration: Drinking lots of clean drinking water throughout the day will help eliminate toxins as well as keep your body well-hydrated.

Lifestyle Practices:

Ayurvedic detoxification includes lifestyle changes which aid in eliminating toxins and overall health. The most important practices are:

Dry-brushing (Garshana) Gentlely applying dry hair prior to showering can increase the flow of lymph and assists in the elimination of the toxins.

The pulling of oil (Gandusha) A process of swirling oil around the mouth for several minutes, usually using coconut or sesame oil.

It assists in eliminating bacteria and toxins and aids in maintaining oral hygiene.

Sauna therapy or steam therapy Affecting sweating with sauna or steam therapy aids in eliminating toxic substances from the skin. It also encourages relaxation.

Exercise regularly: Participating with regular exercise including walking, yoga or aerobic exercise that is moderate aids in lymphatic circulation, flow, and improves the process of detoxification.

Rest and relaxation that is adequate Giving your body enough relaxation and quality rest helps replenish energy levels, strengthen tissues and aids our body's own detoxification process.

Ayurvedic detoxification methods are best done with supervision of an experienced Ayurvedic practitioner to make sure the practices are suitable for your particular constitution and medical needs.

In the next section in the next chapter, we'll look at Ayurvedic herb remedies utilized to help support different aspects of well-being and health.

Ayurvedic herbal Remedies Herbal remedies form essential to Ayurvedic medical practices. In this section we will explore Ayurvedic herbal remedies used throughout the centuries to aid in various aspects of wellness and health. They utilize the healing powers of herbs, medicinal plants and spices in order to correct certain imbalances, improve energy, and restore balance in the mind and body.

Ayurvedic principles of herbal remedies: Ayurvedic herbal remedies are built on the core principle of Ayurveda that include the comprehension of doshas, six taste (rasas) and the benefits of plants. The remedies are adapted to the individual's specific nature (prakriti) as well as imbalances (vikriti) and imbalances (vikriti), with consideration of the particular requirements of each person.

Common Ayurvedic Herbs and Benefits The world is filled with an variety of Ayurvedic herb used in the traditional practice of healing. Below are some of the more commonly used herbs with their advantages:

Ashwagandha (Withania somnifera) is known as an adaptogenic herb ashwagandha can help combat anxiety, improve relaxation and boost overall health. Additionally, it helps boost mental clarity as well as to strengthen your immune system.

Triphala is a combination of three different fruits (amalaki as well as bibhitaki and Haritaki) Triphala is an herbal remedy that is gentle but effective. cure for 29

that aids in promoting digestive health, detoxification, and for promoting digestion, detoxification, and. It balances the doshas, and promotes general health in the gastrointestinal tract.

Turmeric (Curcuma longa): Turmeric is renowned for its anti-inflammatory power and antioxidant capabilities. It helps with digestion, joint health as well as overall health.

Curcumin, which is the main ingredient found in turmeric, is renowned for its many health benefits.

Tulsi (Holy Basil): Tulsi is considered as a sacred plant as part of Ayurveda and is renowned for its properties that aid in adapting. It assists in stress reduction and boosts the immune system and helps improve respiratory health.

Brahmi (Bacopa monnieri): Brahmi is a well-known herb that is used to improve cognition, memory and mental focus. It's often utilized as a brain-tonic that aids in stress and relaxation diminution.

Ginger (Zingiber officinale) Ginger (Zingiber officinale) is a herb that warms you and is that is well-known for its digestive qualities. It helps with digestion, reduces nausea as well as aids in maintaining breathing health. In addition, ginger is used to enhance its anti-inflammatory qualities.

Neem (Azadirachta indica): Neem is a widely used herb for its antifungal, antibacterial blood purifying, and antibacterial properties. It improves skin health and helps to maintain good dental hygiene and encourages elimination.

Guggul (Commiphora mukul): Guggul is a resin that is known for its ability to lower cholesterol levels. It is also beneficial for joints and aids in maintaining the proper weight control.

Licorice (Glycyrrhiza Glabra) Licorice is a herb that has anti-inflammatory and soothing characteristics. It aids in respiration health, relaxes digestion and improves the function of the adrenal glands.

Here are a few examples of the various Ayurvedic herbal remedies. treatment. It is crucial to talk an experienced 30

Ayurvedic specialist or herbalist can identify the best herbal remedies for your specific requirements.

Ayurvedic Herbal Formulations:

In Ayurveda it is common for herbs to be blended to produce potent herbal formulas, called rasayanas or the churnas. They are designed to treat specific imbalances and improve overall health. The most popular Ayurvedic formulas are:

Chyawanprash: Chyawanprash is a replenishing herbal syrup that blends various herbs which include amla (Indian gooseberry) Ashwagandha, amla, and Ghee. It can help improve immunity, improve energy levels, and increase long-term health.

Trikatu Churna: Trikatu churna is a mix made up of three warming spices including black pepper, ginger and long pepper. It assists in digestion, improves metabolism and aids in eliminating the toxins.

Dashmoolarishta: Dashmoolarishta can be described Ayurvedic tonic that is made of 10 herbs. It aids in the balance of Vata dosha, helps support the nervous system and enhances overall health.

Mahasudarshan Churna: Mahasudarshan churna is a blend of herbs designed to strengthen the immune system as well as promote digestive health. It includes herbs like Kutki, neem and Guduchi.

The herbal formulas are typically sold in powder, liquid or tablets. They are prepared with the traditional Ayurvedic methods that ensure the highest effectiveness and potency.

Herbal Remedies for Common Ailments:

Ayurvedic herbal treatments provide safe holistic solutions to treat the most common illnesses. Here are a few instances:

Digestive Problems Herbs like coriander, fennel, and peppermint may help ease digestion-related discomforts, such as bloating as well as indigestion.

Stress and Anxiety Ashwagandha, Brahmi, and Jatamansi are all herbs that have been praised as calming and reduction of stress properties. They can help improve peace, mental clarity and emotional health.

Respiratory Health: Herbs such as the tulsi plant, licorice and eucalyptus can help improve the respiratory system, reduce coughs and clear congestion.

skin health: Neem turmeric and aloe vera are known for their healing qualities. They can help treat different skin issues and encourage healthier skin.

Women's Health Ayurvedic herbaceous substances like the shatavari, ashoka and lodhra can be used to help women maintain their hormone balance, reproductive health and overall well-being during menstrual cycles.

It is crucial to remember that Ayurvedic herb remedies must be taken under the direction by a certified Ayurvedic practitioner. They take into account individual variables like health, constitution, imbalances, as well as any medical conditions that are present.

In the next section we'll look at Ayurvedic solutions for home remedies to treat hair and skin care and provide natural remedies for keeping healthy and glowing hair and skin.

Ayurvedic home Remedies for your Skin and Hair Ayurveda offers a wealth of natural solutions for maintaining radiant and healthy hair and skin. In this section we look at Ayurvedic methods for self-care that harness the healing power of oils, herbs, as well as natural components to help improve healthy hair and skin. The remedies can be simple to cook and can easily be included in your regular regimen of self-care.

Chapter 14: Cleansing And Nourishing The Skin

a. Cleansing:

Besan (Chickpea Flour) Cleanser: Mix besan in a tiny amount of rose water to make an oil. Apply it to the face before washing with warm water.

Besan is a cleanser for the skin. It cleanses the skin, and helps to promote an overall healthy glow.

The Honey Lemon Cleanser Combine equal portions of fresh lemon juice. Apply the mixture to your skin and allow it to stay for about a minute. Cleanse the face with water. This cleanser can help eliminate the excess oil, clear pores, and even out the complexion.

b. Exfoliation:

Ubtan (Herbal Scrub) Make Ubtan by mixing besan and turmeric with coconut powder, sandalwood powder and either rose or milk.

Rub the mix gently onto dry skin and rinse. Ubtan removes dead skin cells and improves the texture of skin, and increases the radiance of your skin.

c. Moisturizing:

Rose Water and Aloe Vera Toner: Mix equal portions of rose water and aloe gel. Apply it on the skin using the help of a cotton pad. The toner will moisturize, soften and even out the pH of your skin.

Almond Oil along with Saffron Face Oil: Mix the almond oil, along with one teaspoon of saffron. Apply the mix to the skin. Almond oil is nourishing and moisturizing the skin while saffron brightens your complexion.

Rejuvenating and Nourishing the Hair:

a. Scalp Massage:

Coconut Oil Scalp Massage: The coconut oil is warm and then gentle massage it on the scalp in circular movements. Allow it to remain on for several days or even overnight prior to washing. The massage on the scalp nourishes hair follicles, improves circulation, and assists in maintaining the health of your scalp.

Ayurvedic Herbal Hair Oil Create a hair oil made from herbs by infusing sesame or coconut oil with various herbs like Brahmi, amla, brahmi and the hibiscus. Massage the oil on hair and scalp, and then let it sit for several days or for a night.

The oil is a natural source of nourishment for the hair and strengthens the hair's roots and encourages healthy hair development.

b. Hair Masks:

Fenugreek and yogurt hair Mask The best way to use it is to soak the seeds of fenugreek for a few hours, and then crush the seeds into a powder. Mix the paste and yogurt before applying it on the locks and the scalp. Apply it for between 30 and 60 minutes before washing. The mask will help condition your hair, prevent dandruff and boosts scalp health.

Aloe Vera and Curry Leaves Hair Mask Blend freshly-made aloe vera gel and curry leaves in order to make an even paste. Apply it to your hair and scalp and let it sit for about 30 minutes prior to washing. The mask is nourishing for hair, increases shine and prevents hair loss.

Herbal tea and infusions to improve skin and Hair Health: a. Green Tea: Consuming green tea on a regular basis gives antioxidant benefits, which help to improve overall skin health, lessen inflammation, and shield from UV damages.

B. Nettle Tea Nettle tea is a great source in vitamins and minerals which help to promote healthy hair growth. improve the health of hair follicles and decrease hair loss.

C. Hibiscus Tea: Hibiscus tea is renowned because of its abundant amount of antioxidants and vitamins which nourish hair, enhance hair health and sparkle to hair.

Lifestyle practices for skin and Hair Health: In conjunction with the solutions above, Ayurveda emphasizes holistic lifestyle methods to maintain good hair and skin health:

Be sure to follow a well-balanced Ayurvedic diet that is based on your body's constitution and imbalances.

Keep hydrated by drinking enough drinking water throughout all whole day.

Use techniques for stress reduction like meditation, yoga and breathing exercises.

Sleep enough to allow your body and mind to refuel.

Keep in mind that patience and consistency are essential to use Ayurvedic natural remedies for your hair and skin care. It's crucial to be aware of the way your hair and skin respond to different treatments and then adjust your regimen according to your individual needs. If you are suffering from specific issues with your hair or skin It is recommended to talk to an Ayurvedic specialist for individualized guidance.

In the next section we'll explore Ayurvedic solutions to the most common illnesses, offering the most natural remedies for different health issues.

Ayurvedic home remedies for common ailments Ayurveda provides a variety of natural cures to treat general ailments and improve overall wellbeing. In this section we will explore Ayurvedic solutions for home use that are easily created and applied to relieve many health problems. The remedies come from spices, herbs along with other organic ingredients they have been employed throughout time to promote the healing process and bring balance back to your body.